THE NURSING SYSTEM
Issues, Ethics, and Politics

THE NURSING SYSTEM
Issues, Ethics, and Politics

Gloria Ferraro Donnelly, R.N., M.S.N.
Director, Nursing Program
La Salle College
Philadelphia, Pennsylvania

Andrea Mengel, R.N., M.S.N.
Assistant Professor of Nursing
Community College of Philadelphia
Philadelphia, Pennsylvania

Doris Cook Sutterley, R.N., M.S.N.
Consultant
La Salle College
Philadelphia, Pennsylvania

With a contribution by Patrick J. Geary, Ph.D.
Professor of History, Princeton University
and Mary C. Geary, R.N., M.S.N.
Formerly, Instructor of Nursing
Trenton State College

A WILEY MEDICAL PUBLICATION
JOHN WILEY & SONS
New York · Chichester · Brisbane · Toronto

Library of Congress Cataloging in Publication Data

Donnelly, Gloria Ferraro.
  The nursing system.

  (A Wiley medical publication)
  Includes index.
    1. Nursing—United States.   I. Mengel, Andrea,
joint author.   II. Sutterley, Doris Cook, joint
author.   III. Title. [DNLM: 1. Philosophy,
Nursing. WY86 D685n]
RT4.D66   610.73   80-12402
ISBN 0-471-04441-5

Printed in the United States of America

10 9 8 7 6 5 4 3 2 1

Preface

The central purpose of this book is to introduce different ways of thinking about the nursing system and its interaction with other systems. In this text we examine the structure and processes of the nursing system as it interacts with other systems, drawing comparisons between the evolution of nursing and other systems.

This book is specifically designed to show nurses that there is more than one method to accomplish an end. The text concentrates primarily on exposing the paradoxes and confusions in the nursing system and in the nursing role as it focuses on issues universally identifiable to nurses. It encourages students to use conflict as a source of growth.

This is not a history book, although it draws on an historical perspective. It is not a manual or workbook, although it contains many exercises designed to challenge the reader's stereotyped notions and idealistic beliefs about the nursing system. It is not a glorification of nursing, although it often emphasizes the creative accomplishments of nursing leaders. It is not a book that pretends to raise every question that needs to be explored in the nursing system, although it raises enough questions to give readers an idea of the complexity of the issues facing nursing.

We have written a process book. We envision nursing students, nursing educators, and practicing nurses sitting in seminars, artfully debating the paradoxical issues treated in this book. The use of metaphor, humor, and the influence of Eastern thinking is intended to structure creative discussion in issues and trends courses as well as in other nursing courses.

We have based much of this text on our own nursing experiences. We express opinions and viewpoints that, at times, may diverge from current popular thinking in nursing, but we do so in order to stimulate thinking, discussion, and debate. We do not presume our viewpoints are always right.

The text is intended for nursing students, practicing nurses suffering from reality shock, and survivors in the system. Other health care professionals who need to know where nursing has been and where it might go may also find the text helpful. Hopefully, the book can become a catalyst for change, as nurses begin to realize that:

> **Reality is only partly our invention; it is also partly our discovery. Our task is to discover how much and in what areas which is which; and then to determine how much new freedom this gives us and what we can do with it.***

Gloria Ferraro Donnelly
Andrea Mengel
Doris Cook Sutterley

*LeShan, Lawrence. *Alternate Realities*. New York, Ballantine Books, 1976.

Contents

THE NURSING SYSTEM
Issues, Ethics, and Politics

CHAPTER **ONE**
The Nursing System

As long as we rest on the security of our certainty, nothing
new can come to us.

A. Low*

NURSING AND THE SISYPHUS SYNDROME

Sisyphus, the clever king in Greek mythology who consistently
outwitted the gods, was forced to spend eternity rolling a huge
stone up a steep hill. Each time Sisyphus approached the summit
of the hill, the weighty stone would roll back to the bottom. And
each time he began the task anew. Punished for his creativity,
Sisyphus persevered in the meaningless activity forced upon him
by the gods. Best to keep Sisyphus busy than to be outwitted
again, reasoned the gods.

Although myth is only a reflection of reality, the story of
Sisyphus is reminiscent of patterns and themes woven into the
history of nursing. Since the origins of formalized nursing in the
Middle Ages, the profession of nursing has been rolling the same
stones up and down the health-care hill. An issue that seems to be
resolved gets reopened, agonized over, and pushed up the hill,
only to roll to the bottom again.

*From reference 2.

ISSUES AS KOANS

Issues in the nursing system are like koans in Zen, which is an Eastern philosophical system. A koan is a nonsensical riddle or a perplexing question posed by a Zen master to his student. The koan is designed to interrupt the thought processes, to reveal the paradoxes inherent in reality, and to force the student into experiencing reality in a different way. The koan is not solved solely by the intellect, although the intellect is involved. Nor does the koan have, in the logical Western sense, a "right" answer. A koan helps a student to gain insight into reality. This insight is reached often after years of struggle with the koan.

To solve a koan one must be "standing at an extremity, with no possibility of choice confronting one. There is just one thing which one must do"(1). This is not to imply that the "just one thing" is the objectively correct course of action, only that the course of action taken is the one that is right for the person choosing it. Margaret Sanger, who began the Planned Parenthood movement, must have experienced this compulsion of choice as she stood over the bed of the dying woman whom she had nursed back to health months before after an illegal abortion. The woman died of a second abortion, and Margaret Sanger vowed to free women from the bonds of biology and to promote birth control as a basic human right. She did this pioneering work without the help of organized nursing. She did not convene a committee. Koans are not solved through committee work.

The struggle with a koan or an issue simultaneously involves the wholeness of the practitioner (the nurse), the dilemma presented, and the problems, worries, and confusions of day-to-day experience. The Zen teacher "uses all his skill to awaken and heighten the profound perplexity, the condition in which the mind is unable to settle on a comforting conclusion and equally unable to forage for a distracting thought"(2). A perusal of nursing issues confirms the fact that there are no comforting conclusions. The resolution of any issue will have its price.

A famous Zen koan is, "What is the sound of one hand clapping?" This question raises the same confusion and puzzlement as the nursing issues, "Who controls nursing practice?" and "How shall nurses be educated?" It could be that the nursing system has not yet struggled enough with these koans to "be standing at an extremity, with no possibility of choice." It is certain that individual nurses are so caught up in dealing with the problems and confusions of daily functions that they do not allow themselves the luxury of or do not have the time to give to struggling with these issues.

Consider the educational system. Florence Nightingale believed that schools of nursing should be "freestanding," that is, independent administratively and economically from the hospital in which they conducted their educational activities. Yet in America the first schools of nursing were attached to hospitals. They were neither economically nor administratively independent of the hospitals' management. In 1905 Adelaide Nutting reiterated Nightingale's stand, saying that schools of nursing should rest on a separate foundation(3). The stone again began to edge up the hill. In 1909, Dr. Richard Olding Beard, of the University of Minnesota, proposed and eloquently defended the university education of nurses in an address given before the American Federation of Nurses (AFN) in St. Paul, Minnesota. His address, entitled "The University Education of the Nurse," warned against beginning the vocational stage of nursing education too soon. He insisted that "the men and women of high rank in any calling . . . have laid broad foundations of knowledge, before they have set their special type of superstructure thereon"(4). The University of Minnesota was one of the first institutions to grant the baccalaureate degree to nurses.

In 1910 Dean James E. Russell of Teacher's College, Columbia University, warned that nursing would never gain professional status with an apprenticeship educational system. In 1913 nursing schools began self-studies of their educational practices and curricula spurred on by the acute shortage of applicants. The stone had rolled down the hill again. Adelaide Nutting, who was chairman of the Education Committee of the National League of Nursing Education in 1913, cited two major conditions that she believed were responsible for declines in nursing applicants during this period: "the long hours of duty and the overemphasis on domestic work"(5). The expanded need for nurses brought about by World War I also exposed these conditions in the nursing education system. A "Standard Curriculum for Nursing Schools" was published by the National League for Nursing Education in 1917, before the onset of World War II. It was a major step in upgrading and broadening nursing education programs.

In 1923 the Rockefeller Foundation published the results of a study on nursing and nursing education in the United States that it had funded beginning in 1918. This study, which is referred to as the Goldmark Report(6), advocated that nursing look to institutions of higher education as its base for the future. Shortly after the publication of this report, the Yale University School of Nursing was opened. However, by 1930 university schools of nursing were still a rarity, since nursing did not receive the massive foundation support that was given to medicine for revamping its educational system after the publication of the results of the Flexner study.

In 1934 the report of the Committee on the Grading of Nursing Schools stressed that professional standards could only be maintained with "a collegiate level of education; an enriched curriculum with more and better theory and less and better practice; a better prepared student body and faculty comparable with those in other professional schools; an organization better fitted to safeguard the professional status and freedom of the school, dominated by neither hospital nor treasury nor nursing traditions and funds adequate to provide for such a school"(7).

In the 1940s the stone again started up the hill, when Esther Lucile Brown published her study *Nursing for the Future,*(8), which once again recommended that nursing move into the mainstream of higher education. The 1950s and 1960s was a time of quietude, until, in 1965, the American Nurses Association (ANA) published its *Position Paper* concerning the educational preparation for nurse practitioners and assistants to nurses. The *Position Paper* again asserted that "The education for all those who are licensed to practice nursing should take place in institutions of higher education"(9).

For various economic and social reasons, many hospital schools of nursing closed after the publication of the *American Nurses' Association Position Paper of 1965*. However, there still remain between three and four hundred hospital schools of nursing. Although the importance of a college education in the sixties may have been a major contributing factor to the closing of many of the hospital schools, the *American Nurses' Association Position Paper on the Educational Preparation for Nurse Practitioners and Assistants to Nurses* did act as a catalyst, bringing us a bit closer to Nightingale's goal of independent schools. The momentum, however, may have been interrupted by the American Nurses'

Association *Statement on Diploma Graduates,* published in 1973 (10). The statement itself was not a retraction of its 1965 position on nursing education but more of an attempt to mollify those nurses without baccalaureate degrees who were concerned about the effects on their professional status if nursing education did move exclusively into the colleges and universities. In light of the fact that it is its membership that keeps an organization intact, it is not difficult to understand the ANA's action in 1973.

In the early 1970s another study of the national nursing scene conducted by J. Lysaught recommended that nursing education make the final move into colleges and universities(11). This goal has yet to be accomplished. A proliferation of associate degree programs in nursing since the 1960s complicates the unresolved koan "How shall nurses be educated?" even further (see Chap. 5).

This koan continues to divide the nursing profession. With all of the studies, reports, and pronouncements of the past one hundred years on the desirability of moving nursing education into the mainstream of higher education, the goal is still not accomplished. In contrast, the medical profession, with solid support from the American Medical Association (AMA), revamped its entire medical education system relatively soon (thirty years) after the publication of the Flexner Report (see Chap. 5 for details).

Neither the nursing system nor the medical system has developed in isolation of the social, economic, and political climates of the times. No doubt economic factors will finally cause the closing of hospital schools of nursing as third-party payers such as health insurers become increasingly reluctant to commit health insurance dollars to financing nursing education. However, the evolution of nursing education is illustrative of nursing's lack of control over its own destiny.

Nutting and Lavinia Dock, who worked for women's suffrage early in the twentieth century, in their four-volume history of nursing(12) referred to nursing's interdependence with other systems. "Only in the light of history can she [the nurse] clearly see how closely her own calling is linked with the general conditions of education and of liberty that obtain—as they rise, she rises, and as they sink, she falls"(12). Thus, Nutting and Dock considered the nursing profession not as its own prime mover but as a system that interacts with and is in large part shaped by the forces and changes in other systems such as the medical system, the hospital system, the political system, and the economic system, and that is strongly influenced by the role of women in society.

THE PURPOSE OF THE NURSING SYSTEM

Nursing can be conceptualized as a system. A system is a set of components constantly interacting with one another to form a whole that transcends and differs from the sum of its parts. Nursing is a system created by people to serve a purpose. To understand the purpose is to understand the essence of the system. The purpose of the nursing system has not yet been clearly defined and often changes as a result of the conceptions of people outside the system.

Early in nursing's history, religious influences largely shaped the purpose of nursing. Formal nursing from the fifth to the seventeenth centuries was dominated in Europe by religious communities including the Benedictines, the Augustinian Sisters, the Franciscan Friars, and the Sisters of Charity—the oldest nursing order of nuns in existence. One of the original motivations for caring for the sick was to insure one's salvation by engaging in self-sacrificing works. Today, altruism—a desire to help others—has replaced salvation as the motivating factor in choosing nursing as a career.

KOAN

List, in order of importance, five reasons for choosing nursing as your career.

1. _____

2. _____

3. _____

4. _____

5. _____

> Is there a balance between altruism, lofty inten-
> tions, and your own needs for security and self-
> actualization, and a desire to contribute to the ad-
> vancement of the nursing profession?

To insure their own salvation and to encourage the salvation of others, the religious orders cared for the sick in great monastic hospitals until the Protestant Reformation in the sixteenth century. Hospital conditions and nursing standards generally deteriorated after the Reformation, when unkempt, untrained secular nurses dominated the hospital scene, especially in England, while the nurses from religious orders were overworked and hampered by strict rules of modesty. A dichotomy of function began to evolve as the religious nurses increasingly tended to the patient's soul and the "Sairey Gamps," (unkempt, drunken nurses, such as the one in Dickens' novel) tended the body, which in many orthodox religious philosophies was believed to be corrupt. Woodham-Smith(13) in a discussion of the divergent perceptions of the functions of the nurse in the 1800s, said, "Amongst women who were prepared to devote themselves to the sick, there were two totally different conceptions of the functions of a nurse. The hospital nurse, drunken, promiscuous, and troublesome, considered that her function was to tend her patient's sick body and to restore him to physical health by carrying out the doctor's orders. The religious orders, sisters and nuns, were neither drunken nor promiscuous, but were apt to be more concerned with the souls of their patients than with their bodies"(13). Florence Nightingale might have believed that the two functions—caring for the body and caring for the soul—were complementary when she referred to nursing as a "calling." An overemphasis on one to the exclusion of the other, which Nightingale found unacceptable, creates an imbalance in the nursing role and confusion concerning nursing's purpose.

Current dissension over the purpose and definition of nursing centers around the nurse's assumption of more and more physician's duties in the expanded role as "physician extenders." Debate in the early years of this century focused on a very different issue—the importance of nurses assuming maids' duties when the households in which they practiced private-duty nursing had a shortage of help. The following letter to the editor of the *American Journal of Nursing* in 1908(14) illustrates the confusion over the purpose of nursing.

AN OLD QUESTION ASKED ANEW

Dear Editor: Just what is required of the nurse in the private home? Recently an article in the *New York Sun* attracted my attention. "A chance for a new calling, that opens a profitable field for young women; great need for working nurses who will do the little things that the trained nurse sniffs at," is the way the article is headed and which goes on to say that the regular trained nurse of to-day absolutely refuses to sweep or dust her patient's room, from the fact that she cannot do menial labor, and that if asked to perform some slight or trivial service she appears positively shocked.

Is this true? I, for one, in the great body of graduate nurses, feel that it is not, and while I do not for a minute think of us as taking the place of a servant, I do feel that we, as a body of intelligent women, have too much good *common sense* or *mother wit* to retard the recovery of our patients by allowing them to worry over little things left undone oftentimes, which we could do easily, and without lowering our dignity in the least.

Of the many nurses with whom I am personally acquainted, I am sure there is not one who would hesitate for an instant to clean her patient's room, not only one day but every day, if necessary.

I am now in a home where there are four cases of typhoid. There are three nurses here, but we do not clean the rooms because the people have five servants and do not want us to do so. Of course in this instance it is not necessary, but in a very great number of homes to which I am called, I do clean my room.

I was in a home last year where the mother was quite ill, and beside caring for her constantly, I dressed three little girls for school, bathing them, combing their hair and making the necessary toilet each morning; ordered the groceries and managed the house in general, there being only one servant (she was new), so there was no one else to do these little things.

I think that we as nurses try to conform to whatever conditions we meet, and as far as possible adapt ourselves to the needs of the homes in which we daily find ourselves. I believe I voice the sentiment of the nurses of "Sunny Tennessee." I would like to have the opinion of others on this question, especially from some of the New York nurses, since the article to which I refer was suggested by a woman who "conducts one of the high-class employment bureaus of West Side, New York," so the paper states.

If this really is true, is it any wonder some of the doctors do not appreciate and patronize "graduates" more fully and exclusively?

This letter to the editor appeared in the American Journal of Nursing, Volume VIII, No. 11, August, 1908, p. 925–925

The nurse who wrote the letter was troubled by the fact that "trained" nurses were asserting their right to divorce the nursing role from domestic chores and to more fully define nursing functions. For centuries nurses have tried to "conform to whatever conditions they met," perhaps because the work and the concept of nursing has been so intertwined with the concept of the traditional female role. Nutting and Dock point out that the word *nursing* was originally used to mean "the nurture and care of the well child" and later to mean "relief and care of the sick and infirm." Their model of nursing (Fig. 1-1) is certainly a visionary one.

Dock and Stewart (3, p. 355) wrote in 1938 that the purpose of nursing is *to promote and conserve health and prevent disease; protect and care for peoples' social and physical environment; and care for the whole person, mind and body.* To achieve this purpose, Dock and Stewart advocated a broad-based scientific education and research-oriented practice. "Nurses," they said, ". . . are becoming increasingly active not only as consumers but as producers of knowledge. The field is full of problems that need scientific study. . . . No one will question the responsibility of the nurse for improving the reliability and effectiveness of her own procedures. . . . Indeed the art of nursing would be blind and helpless—even dangerous—without the guidance of science"(3, p. 358).

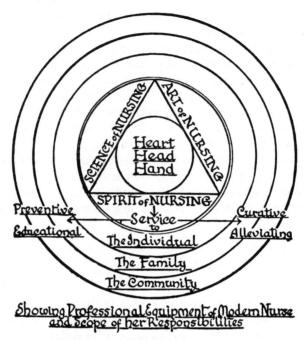

Figure 1-1.
(Reproduced with permission [12])

This view of nursing's purpose, written in 1938, is as accurate today as it was when it was written. However, many other systems and forces have mediated against this view of nursing's purpose. For example, in 1901 the *Journal of the American Medical Association* carried an editorial entitled "The Unsentimental Nurse."* The writer asserted that some physicians found the "trained" nurse to be "conceited and too unconscious of the due subordination she owes to the medical profession, *of which she is a sort of useful parasite***"(15). Those who endured the ministrations of this trained nurse, the editorial continued, often objected to "her noiseless efficiency, her conscientious regularity, her simulated amiability, her mechanical perfection in the performance of duties, her emotional impassibility." The editorial

---

*The word *unsentimental* refers to what may be the end result of exposing a nurse to too much scientific education. The implication is that an increase in knowledge is directly proportionate to a decrease in empathy.

**Present authors' italics.

ended on a patronizing note: "When a nurse can, with all her other requirements met, steer clear of the Scylla of emotionalism on the one hand and the Charybdis of indifference on the other, she is a wonderful creature, common as she may be and then if she is still criticized one ought to love her for the enemies she has made"(15, p. 33).

Is nursing, then, a domesticated, humanistic branch of scientific medicine? Is nursing's central purpose to assume those duties delegated by physicians as technology broadens the scope of specialized medical practice?

Nursing has always filled the voids left by shortages in personnel as physicians and other health professionals have moved into new arenas and bequeathed "routine" duties and tasks to nursing. For example, an issue involving the use of nurses as private surgical assistants to physicians has been debated recently by the American Association of Operating Room Nurses (AORN). A special committee of AORN reported that these nurses are practicing in a "physician extender" role, and that this practice cuts down on the time spent in direct patient care. However, the delegates to AORN's convention rejected the special committee's report, concluding that private surgical assistants are practicing nursing. "If nurses don't assume the role of first assistant," says a nurse in OR inservice education, "then it's going to fall to less trained, less qualified technicians who wouldn't have knowledge of the principles behind surgery. . . ."(16). Such situations pose a dilemma for a profession whose members are so thoroughly programmed into feeling responsible for finding solutions to all problems presented. The primary focus of concern should not be on a particular task or function but on the much broader issue of whether or not the nursing profession determines and pursues new roles and responsibilities on its own initiative, or waits for a crisis to occur or for directions from others to fill a void. In its continued efforts to respond to all needs, the nursing system itself has created barriers to the ultimate defining of its purpose.

Definitions of nursing may make pronouncements about the nature of nursing. However, any system that is in dynamic interaction with other systems can have no static purpose, "for purpose is a relation, not a thing to have"(17). A system, any system, represents the point of view of one or several observers. Therefore, relationships or boundaries between systems must be taken into consideration in order to understand the dilemma of purpose.

Table 1-1 shows how several nursing leaders have viewed the purpose of nursing. Compare your view with those of the leaders presented.

KOAN

Three nursing elders walked through a meadow searching for enlightenment on the purpose of nursing. The first said that the ultimate purpose of nursing was to care for the sick and suffering. The second asserted that the ultimate purpose of nursing was to assist the physician in his sacred work. The third reported that it was revealed in a vision that the ultimate purpose of nursing is to advance the health of all peoples and contribute to knowledge in the science of man.

How would you answer the elders?

TERRITORIES AND BOUNDARIES

When the purpose of a system is generally agreed upon, at least by a majority of the people who function within it, a vying for territory begins by those within the system and those outside of it. The territory, for purposes of discussing the nursing system, is the behavior space of a person acting in the nursing role. Territory in nursing is synonymous with role.

Analogies can be drawn from ethological studies on the territorial behavior of animals. A territory's value is dervied from its position. Central territories have higher value. For example, an animal who establishes a territory in a sheltered nest at the center of the jungle will have greater success in defending against attackers than one who moves about on the periphery like a nomad. Perhaps, because of confusion over purpose, nursing seems to operate on the periphery of the health care delivery system, easily slipping into other roles or territories as demands dictate. This is especially evident in many hospital systems,

Table 1–1.   Views on the Purpose of Nursing

Nursing Leaders	Statement of Purpose of Nursing
Florence Nightengale —1859 (18)	To put the patient in the best condition for nature to act upon him.
Lavinia Dock and Isabel Stewart —1938 (3, p. 355)	To promote and conserve health and prevent disease; protect and care for people's social and physical environment and care for the whole person, mind and body.
Dorothy Johnson —1959 (19)	To assist the patient in the maintenance or re-establishment of a moving state of equilibrium throughout the health change process.
Virginia Henderson —1964 (20)	To assist the individual, sick or well, in the performance of those activities contributing to health or its recovery (or to peaceful death) that he would perform unaided if he had the necessary strength, will or knowledge and to do this in such a way as to help him gain independence as rapidly as possible.
Sister Madeleine Clemence Vaillot —1966 (21)	To help the patient become an "authentic person" and to use his situation, the illness, for doing so.
Martha Rogers —1970 (22)	To help people achieve their maximum health potential. Nursing's first line of defense is promotion of health and prevention of illness. Care of the sick is resorted to when our first line of defense fails.

where nurses often assume the roles of pharmacists, lab technicians, or ward secretaries on evening or night shifts.

This lack of a central role in nursing is also evident in the
"physician extender" roles that have been evolving recently.

KOAN

**A nurse and a physician working in a neighbor-
hood health clinic had finished their work for the
day. The nurse, who enjoyed the independence
and challenge of the job, said to the physician, "It
is such a delight to work in an expanded nursing
role." The physician looking puzzled said, "But
you are not an expanded nurse, you are a physician extender!"**

How would you resolve this dilemma?

The territories of nursing and medicine within the environment
of the health care delivery system have always been a source of
confusion and conflict. Which of the following models symbolizes
the relationship between the territories of nursing and medicine
in today's health care system?

The model in Figure 1-2 which incorporates nursing within the

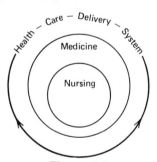

Figure 1-2.

realm of medicine's territory, is a commonly held view. Revised Nurse Practice Acts have made this model largely inoperative except in those instances when nursing assumes a role or a function traditionally carried out by medicine. Many health care agencies, particularly hospitals, have failed to recognize this model as obsolete.

The model in Figure 1-3 in which medicine and nursing are two distinct territories within the health care system, is a newer model that is strongly supported by the nursing leadership. This model illustrates that medicine and nursing are separate and different services and collaborate. In the gray or overlapping areas they negotiate. In this model, the leader of the team is defined by the nature of the problem.

The model in Figure 1-4 developed by an innovative nursing

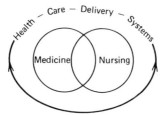

Figure 1-3.

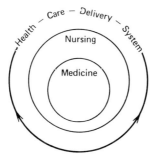

Figure 1-4.

student in a baccalaureate program course on issues,* illustrates that the highly technical territory of medicine is a part of the larger holistic territory of nursing. Cure-oriented medicine is but a small part of care-oriented nursing. This may be a very futuristic model of the relationship between nursing and medicine; however, even in this model, medicine can retain control of nursing just as the nucleus of a cell controls and coordinates the rest of the cell.

KOAN

Develop your own model of how you perceive the relationship between the territories of medicine and nursing.

The boundary of a territory or role is delineated by the decisions that can be made within the role(2, p.131). "To define the boundaries of a role it is simply necessary to determine what decisions can be made in that role. However, a boundary cannot be a boundary in isolation. Little purpose is served by simply establishing the decision boundaries of one role. It is also necessary to establish the decision boundaries of roles that juxtapose, and this juxtaposition will be brought about through the interaction of task cycles"(2, p. 131).

This concept of using the parameters of decision-making to define boundaries creates even more dilemmas within and beyond the nursing system boundaries. In most hospital systems, for example, the director of nursing is organizationally and legally (since a director can be sued for hiring a negligent person or one without proper credentials) responsible for the hiring and firing of members of the nursing staff, except in cases where special units in the hospital are decentralized from the nursing department and operate autonomously with their own budget and administration. Physicians in many hospitals, however, have en-

---

*L. Beardsley, a student at Trenton State College, New Jersey Department of Nursing, Spring 1978.

joyed informal input into the hiring, promotion, and firing of members of the nursing staff even though, technically, this kind of decision-making is not within their role-territory. Consider the following case.

It would seem logical that the best qualified person be chosen for a nursing coordinator position in a specialty unit of a medical center. In one situation, judgment concerning what constituted the best qualifications precipitated a divisive and bitter argument between the chief physician of the unit and the director of nursing, who was legally and administratively responsible for the practice of nursing in that unit. The director of nursing chose Ms. Green on the basis of her nursing experience, educational background, and management abilities. The physician argued loudly and unpleasantly at meetings and in memos that he be permitted to "champion his candidate" for the position. He wanted Ms. Blue to be appointed because he was better able to work with her. He viewed the director of nursing's refusal to rescind Ms. Green's appointment as a display of obstinacy and hostility rather than as an administrative perogative. The hospital administrator backed the director of nursing's right to decide, but the physician launched a fierce negative campaign against the director of nursing that ultimately led to her dismissal.

Because physicians generalize their expertise and authority to other than just medical affairs and because a large number of nurses has accepted this intrusion, boundary skirmishes between the two systems are likely to continue.

Boundaries between the subsystems in nursing are often quite confusing as well. For example, what decisions can a registered nurse (RN) make that a licensed practical nurse (LPN) cannot make? Is there a consistent and well-defined range of decision-making for each level in the nursing hierarchy? Use Table 1-2 to help you analyze the pattern and scope of decision-making in each of the nursing subsystems. Sometime in the course of your clinical experience in one institution, ask each type of nurse listed in the decision table to give you the following information: "Give specific examples of the kinds of decisions you make in your role

Table 1-2. Decision Table

Nurse Administrator or Director of Nursing	Supervisor or Coordinator	Head Nurse	Staff Nurse	Clinical Specialist	Primary Nurse	LPN or LVN

as _____ in the course of a week." List the decisions under the appropriate heading. Then examine the overlap, the duplication of effort, and the differentiation in each nursing subrole.

HIERARCHIES AND PECKING ORDERS

Hierarchies are evident in every complex living system, and the nursing system is no exception. The term *hierarchy* evokes different images in different people. Some hierarchies are horizontal, although that is not the way hierarchies in nursing are usually conceptualized. Horizontal hierarchies are most evident in organizations in which there is a strong equalized knowledge base among its members or workers. For example, a group practice organization, owned and operated by several physician/specialists, would use a horizontal hierarchy. The primary decision maker or authority in a particular situation would be defined or dictated by the nature of the problem presented by the consumer (see Fig. 1-5).

As nursing broadens its knowledge base, its members seem less satisfied working in the vertical hierarchies that still predominate. The system of nursing care delivery called primary nursing is an example of a horizontal hierarchy in nursing. Each primary nurse is responsible for a case load of patients from admission to discharge. The attending physician consults with the primary nurse assigned to the patient, not with the head nurse. Managerial functions of the unit are often carried out by a unit manager who has no line authority over the primary nurse. The primary nursing care delivery system is based on the premise that the primary nurse has the knowledge and skills to manage the nursing care of a caseload of patients and to be directly accountable for that care.

Horizontal Hierarchy

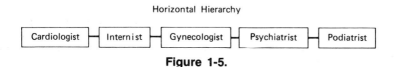

Figure 1-5.

Most nursing departments* within hospital systems still use the vertical hierarchy as their pattern of organization, as shown in Figure 1-6.

The vertical hierarchical pattern of organization originated in the seventeenth century in military organizations and was adopted later by early industrial organizations made up primarily of unskilled laborers. It guaranteed that each person in the system had one boss who had "undisputed power over the subordinate and could therefore force him, by threat of dismissal and loss of his livelihood and self-esteem to toe the line"(2, p. 69). This pattern of organization tends to work best when a system is threatened with deterioration or annihilation, such as an army, or in a system where most of the workers need constant and direct supervision of their activities to ensure that the work is done within a specific time frame, such as supervision of a harvest.

Vertical hierarchies within nursing systems often deteriorate into pecking orders as members at the higher levels of the pyramid begin to feel superior to those with lower rank. (Any rank order hierarchical system promotes this kind of thinking, despite the personalities involved.) The problem is further compounded when the feeling of superiority is generalized to all areas of decision-making instead of to a particular area of expertise.

A nursing administrator with only superficial knowledge in coronary care nursing hired a clinical specialist to pioneer a program in patient teaching, cardiac rehabilitation, and on-going staff development for the coronary care nursing staff. The clinical specialist quickly established herself in the role and with the support of the coronary care medical staff and nursing staff initiated several innovative programs. At her second quarterly evaluation conference with the director of nursing, she detailed her progress and accomplishments to date. She inquired into the possibility of more funding for another project. The director of nursing listened quietly, praised the accomplishments, but remarked at the end of the conference, "I hope you are not

*Not all nursing departments use as high a vertical hierarchy as the one depicted. Many nursing departments are experimenting with flattening out the organizational pyramid and centralizing decision-making authority in the primary nurse, where it is most effective.

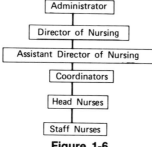

Figure 1-6.

going too far with all of these changes. Don't you think you should check with me in the future before proceeding any further?" The clinical specialist, who was quite used to functioning independently but within the limits of the role description, innocently replied, "I thought I was proceeding in the direction toward which I was hired to go. With my knowledge and experience in coronary care, I certainly felt secure in my decisions and have modified my plans and actions as needed." The director of nursing was visibly annoyed and considered the clinical specialist's reply bordering on insubordination. Both the director and the clinical specialist were caught in the vertical hierarchy trap.

Nursing students and their instructors often get caught in the same trap, particularly when the student is very bright and feels comfortable about asking questions and engaging in dialogue and when the instructor is operating under the *false* assumption that in the student-teacher hierarchy teachers always know more than students.

Nurses who attended very traditional nursing schools often reminisce about the rituals of submission to upperclass students that they went through in order to be integrated into the hierarchical structure of the nursing school.

A nurse who was attending an assertiveness training course recounted her traumatic initiation experiences as a first-year nursing student. She was given directions to polish all of the upperclass students' white shoes for a week, but on the final day she rebelled and polished the

**white shoes both inside and out (creative rebellion). She
was socially ostracized by the nursing student body for several months until the matter was forgotten.**

Such practices, which might be compared to initiation ceremonies
in college fraternities and sororities, are very rare today. However, there still exist some subtle but powerful indoctrination
rituals that are indigenous to the specific setting in which nurses
are educated and in which they practice.

Another drawback to vertical hierarchies is the fact that
creativity is often simultaneously sought after and then suppressed, as in the case of the clinical specialist. A creative person
disrupts the status quo and can become a scapegoat at any level in
the hierarchy.

Vertical hierarchy with its value connotations also influences
how the nursing system views tasks and functions. In a letter to
the editor of a Philadelphia newspaper, a physician explained his
support for the evolving role of the Physician's Assistant category
of health care worker (*The Evening Bulletin,* February 4, 1975, p.
4). The value of the physician's assistant, he said, would be to free
the physician from some of the routine tasks just as the practical
nurse has freed the "R.N. for higher levels of nursing function."
The nurse who practices as a midwife or a family nurse practitioner is often categorized as one who frees the physician for
more complex tasks. The question then becomes how is "higher
functioning" defined? How does the nursing system assign value
to function? Are tasks with greater technological involvement
"higher functions" than tasks involving primarily interpersonal
skills? Do nurses working in intensive care units function on a
higher level than mental-health or psychiatric nurses working in
a community mental health center? Do nurses who work on a
surgical unit function on a higher level than nurses in a nursing
home?

KOAN

**Which of the following activities do you think is
most indicative of "high-level functioning" in
nursing practice?**

1. Giving a complete bed bath with range-of-motion exercise and proper positioning for a patient who has had a recent cerebral vascular accident.
2. Interpreting correctly an electrocardiogram and giving the coronary care patient an emergency drug.
3. Conducting a nursing assessment on a new adult health clinic client.
4. Giving cardiopulmonary resuscitation to an accident victim on your way home from work.
5. Working as a mental-health counselor on a hot-line in a suicide prevention center.

The pecking orders of function and rank that have evolved out of an overuse of vertical hierarchical organization have been divisive to the entire nursing system. Horizontal hierarchies, where differences in expertise are recognized and respected, may begin to heal the divisions.

THE NURSING SYSTEM AS A SET

Any system is made up of a set of members or objects that have characteristics in common. It would be impossible to examine all the members of the "set" of nurses and deduce their common characteristics. Therefore, a set is often represented by a "typical member." "This method rests on the assumption that the set can be typified, an idea that goes back at least to Plato. Platonists argued that the ideal type is a better representation of the set than any enumeration would be, since the actual members of a set could, at best, be faulty realizations of the ideal type"(17, p. 64).

KOAN

Nurse A. is giving Mr. Jones a bed bath. Nurse B. works out of Community Mental Health Center doing Crisis Intervention. Nurse C. is an administrator in a large nursing department. Nurse D. is in private practice as a health counselor. Nurse E. is teaching in a university. Nurse F. conducts staff development programs in a nursing home. Nurse G. delivers babies in the hills of Kentucky.

Who, then, is a typical nurse?

The word *nurse* conjures up many images: a lady in white, an angel of mercy, a professional person. It is very difficult to describe a typical member of the nurse set since different people have divergent viewpoints about what is to be typified. Consider the typical nurse as presented in the media. It is mainly a woman who works in a hospital, wears a white uniform and a cap, and hovers around a nurses' station desk. The nurse in the media is most often typified as being directly responsible to and handmaiden to the physician. The chief nurse in the television series M*A*S*H is a notable exception. The M*A*S*H nurse wields considerable authority with a military bearing over "her nurses." She is not quite a "handmaiden" but rather portrays an aggressive, sometimes scheming, often hysterical, authoritarian woman. There has been minimal focus in the media on the nurse as a skilled and learned professional.

In the past, and in many cases even now, the characterization of the nursing set was often related primarily to external traits and trappings. Consider the actual case in the following Koan that directly relates to equating the external "image" of nurse to the concept of professional.

KOAN

In a small community hospital, the nursing department changed the dress code by offering its nurses the option of wearing caps. Many of the nurses took advantage of the option and stopped wearing caps. One physician announced to a group of nurses that despite the urgency of the situation, he would only speak to nurses who wore caps. To resolve this dilemma, the nurses kept a supply of coffee filters at the desk. When they needed to communicate with this doctor, they would pin on a coffee filter. How do you view their resolution of this dilemma?

Discuss with your peers or colleagues all of the associations the word professional brings to mind when applied to nursing. Develop a statement in answer to the question, "What makes a nurse a professional?"

Have you focused on the externals of uniforms, caps, and pins; on protocol and deportment; on cool, efficient, nonemotional behavior; on ambition and drive; on research and inquiry; on continued pursuit of knowledge? Proceed to the next Koan.

KOAN

Can the nursing set be characterized as professional? Listed below are seven criteria of a profession. After your readings and discussions, indicate next to each criterion whether you believe the nursing system meets that criterion of a profession, then decide if nursing is a profession.

_____ A profession has a constantly enlarging, well-defined body of specialized knowledge that it uses and expands following the scientific method.

_____ A profession educates its members in institutions of higher learning.

_____ A profession applies its body of knowledge to vital social services.

_____ A profession functions autonomously in developing professional policy and controlling professional activity.

_____ A profession attracts individuals who value service and recognize their chosen occupation as a life-work.

> _____ A profession attempts to provide freedom of action, opportunity for continued professional growth, and economic security for its members.
>
> _____ A profession takes responsibility for continued learning.
>
> Is the state of the nursing system professional, semiprofessional, or nonprofessional?

THE STATES OF THE NURSING SYSTEM

Weinberg(17, p. 87) tells us that systems exhibit state-determined behavior. A state is a condition, situation, or pattern that can be recognized if it occurs again. It is difficult to describe definitively the state of the nursing system at present except to say that there are many indicators that the system is in a state of flux or redefinition. One such indicator is the changing labels in nursing. "During and after a revolution things are often renamed to change thinking patterns. . . . In France, in the nineteenth century, _queen bee_ was changed to _laying bee_ as part of the effort to expunge all records of royalty"(17, p. 74). After Henry VIII of England closed the monastic hospitals in England and laicized hospitals, there was an attempt to change the term _Sister_ (head of a hospital ward) to one with no ecclesiastical connotations. The attempt failed because of public sentiment and to this day head nurses in England are still called Sisters(3, pp. 94-96). Recently, the term for _nurse_ in the Rural Clinics Bill was changed from _physician extender_ to _primary care provider_ after testimony by a former president of the ANA, Anne Zimmerman(23). So many new labels have evolved for nurses practicing in what seem to be new roles: nurse practitioner, family nurse clinician, pediatric nurse associate, primary care nurse, clinical specialist. Are these changing labels an indication of the nursing system's state of expansion or state of confusion?

KOAN

List the various titles and names accorded nurses in health care settings in which you learn or work. Classify these names or titles according to whether their meaning relates to function, status in a hierarchy, or relationship to other professionals. Which is the dominant classification? Speculate on the reasons for your findings.

At the opening address of almost every American Nurses' Association Convention the president of the association has invariably stated in some form or another, "This is a most exciting time to be a nurse." One could conclude from this recurrent remark that the state of system also depends upon the viewpoint of the observer. The view from the top of the nursing organization must indeed seem exciting. At the same time, in courses on nursing trends and issues, across the country, students and professors were examining the chaotic state of the nursing education system and the changing state of the practice system. One can assume that the term *exciting* is broad enough to encompass *chaotic* and *changing*.

In Chapter 2, a close look at the organized complexity that characterizes the nursing system and the larger health care delivery system may further illuminate the present and future state of the nursing system.

REFERENCES

1. Suzuki DT: *The Field of Zen*. New York, Harper and Row Publishers Inc, 1969, p. 10.

2. Low A: *Zen and Creative Management*. New York, Anchor Books, 1976, p 201.

3. Stewart I: *The Education of Nurses*. New York, MacMillan Inc, 1944, p 172–173.

4. Beard RO: The university education of the nurse. *Teachers College Record* XI, pp 27–40, 1910.

5. Stewart I: *The Education of Nurses*. New York, Macmillan Inc, 1944, p 189.

6. Goldmark J: *Nursing and Nursing Education in the United States*. New York, Macmillan Inc, 1923.

7. Stewart I: *The Education of Nurses*. New York, Macmillan Inc, 1944, pp 214–215.

8. Brown EL: *Nursing for the Future*. New York, Russell Sage Foundation, 1948.

9. *A Position Paper: Educational Preparation for Nurse Practitioners and Assistants to Nurses*. New York, American Nurses Association, 1965, p 5.

10. Statement on diploma graduates, New York, American Nurses Association, 1973.

11. Lysaught J: *An Abstract for Action*. New York, McGraw Hill Inc, 1970.

12. Nutting A, Dock L: *A History of Nursing, Volume I*. New York, GP Putnams Sons, 1907, p 5.

13. Woodham-Smith C: *Florence Nightingale*. New York, McGraw Hill Inc, 1951, p 93.

14. An old question asked anew: Letter to the editor. *Am J Nurs* 8:924–925, 1908.

15. The unsentimental nurse, Editorial. *JAMA*. 37:33, 1901.

16. Nursing news. *RN* 41:16, 1978.

17. Weinberg GM: *An Introduction to General Systems Thinking*. New York, John Wiley & Sons Inc, 1975, p 57.

18. Nightingale F: *Notes on Nursing*. Philadelphia, JB Lippincott Company, 1946, (facsimile of 1859 edition).

19. Johnson DE: A philosophy of nursing. *Nurs Outlook* 7:198–200, 1959.

20. Henderson V: The nature of nursing. *Am J Nurs* 64:62–68, 1964.

21. Vaillot MC, Sr: Existentialism: A philosophy of commitment. *Am J Nurs* 66:500–505, 1966.

22. Rogers M: *The Theoretical Basis of Nursing Practice.* Philadelphia, FA Davis Company, 1970.

23. Primary care provider substituted as wording in rural clinics bill. *Am J Nurs* 77:1381, 1396, 1977.

CHAPTER TWO

Organized Complexity

In general, we can say that the larger the system becomes, the more parts interact, the more difficult it is to understand environmental constraints, the more obscure becomes the problem of what resources should be made available, and deepest of all, the more difficult becomes the problem of the legitimate values of the system.

C. West Churchman*

THE HEALTH CARE SYSTEM

The American health care system, of which nursing is a large subsystem, is one of the largest industries in the nation. The health care system used to be refered to as a service; now it is called an industry. Changes in the focus of the health care system are evidenced by its characterization as an industry. This recent development accurately reflects the system's change of focus from an altruistic model, which emphasized the goal of serving others, to an egoistic model, which emphasizes the survival of the system itself. For example, the purpose of the hospital, as viewed by the nursing system, is caring for the sick and improving the health

*Churchman CW: Epilogue. The past's future: estimating trends by systems theory, in Kur G (ed): *Trends in General System Theory,* New York, Wiley Interscience, 1971, p 438.

and welfare of the community. However, from the point of view of other systems, a hospital exists for many other reasons: as a source of employment for the community, as a physician's workshop, as a learning laboratory for students of various disciplines, and as a major consumer of equipment and supplies. The full impact of the change from a service model to an industrial model is now being felt by nurses who are being educated in the altruistic, humanistic model. Can conflicts between these two models be resolved? Can nurses be comfortable working in a cost-conscious industry?

KOAN

What reasons do you see for a hospital system to exist? What do you believe is the central purpose of the health care system from the point of view of different groups, including nurses, patients, physicians, social workers, and hospital administrators?

The health care industry has become more conscious of costs recently as a result of scrutiny from systems that pay many of their bills, particularly the government and third-party insurers. According to a major third-party insurer, costs are rising for the following reasons:

· Expansive medical technology. Equipment quickly becomes obsolete and the cost of skilled personnel to operate equipment is high.
· Inappropriate use of services. More emphasis is needed on ambulatory and outpatient care.
· Excessive hospital beds. An oversupply of beds results in pressures that lead to unnecessary admissions and prolonged stays.
· Defensive medicine. Physicians are overdiagnosing and overtreating out of fear of malpractice suits.
· Institution productivity. Technology in hospitals does not mean increased employee productivity. Further, it is recognized that hospitals could be more efficient.

Insurance and federal government programs. These programs have provided reimbursement primarily for inpatient services, leaving few incentives for developing outpatient care programs(1).

The federal government did not get involved in health care until the early twentieth century as a result of preparation for World War I, when one-third of the men called for military service were unable to pass the entrance physical examination. During Franklin Roosevelt's New Deal years, the government was involved in health care as a contributor of funds to state treasuries for health programs, and as a builder of health care facilities through its public works program. After World War II, the American Hospital Association suggested that the federal government get involved in hospital construction, and in 1946 Congress enacted the Hill-Burton Program, which provided funds for hospital construction, education of physicians and nurses, and tighter controls over food and drugs. In 1966 the federal government created regional medical programs to facilitate the sharing of new knowledge about cardiovascular disease and cancer in an effort to decrease the morbidity and mortality of these diseases. The Comprehensive Health Planning Law was enacted the following year to plan for health care "without interfering with existing patterns of private professional practice of medicine, dentistry, and related healing arts"(1, p. 19). These first ventures into the private health care system by the federal government were loosely organized and posed no threat to private practitioners.

In 1974 a federal law was enacted that had the potential to have a major impact on the private sector. The Health Planning and Resources Development Act, Public Law 93-641, was designed to deal with health resources and health planning. The law created health service areas throughout the country. Each area is served by a Health Systems Agency (HSA) that is governed by a board composed of 51 to 60% consumers. The other members of each HSA board are health care providers—nurses, physicians, dentists, and so on. Although the boards are elected by citizen-members of the HSA, the agencies are still quasi-government institutions, since the guidelines under which the agencies function are established by the federal and state governments. The purposes of the HSAs include: to improve the health of residents of the area; to increase the accessibility, acceptability, continuity, and quality of services; to restrict increases in the cost of providing services; and to prevent unnecessary duplication of health resources. Current planning now emphasizes cost containment through a decrease in the number of hospital inpatient beds and an increase in the use of ambulatory and outpatient services. Underused inpatient beds increase costs because unfilled beds cost almost as much as filled beds in terms of fixed costs such as staffing, maintenance, and utilities. These costs are passed on to consumers. Furthermore, unfilled beds may result in unnecessary hospitalization for a variety of reasons in order to use the beds.

HSAs have been invested with a great deal of responsibility and authority. Acceptance of the authority of HSAs is not absolute and success of the planning process established by *The Health Planning and Resources Development Act* cannot be judged at this time. It may be as inadequate as previous attempts to influence health care or it may be the precursor of national health insurance. Providers dissatisfied with HSA rulings on their requests for approval to expand their services or to develop new services have mechanisms for appeal outside of the HSA organizational structure where HSA decisions can be overturned.

Why is the government involved in health care? It is involved for a variety of social, political, and economic reasons. In recent years, Americans have begun to view health care as a fundamental right rather than as a service for those who can afford it. Private citizens, politicians, and federal bureaucrats, concerned with rising costs and increasingly vocal complaints about decreasing services, have been calling for a massive study and a major overhaul of the health care system. The private sector is either unwilling or unable to commit resources to this monumental task.

In earlier years, philanthropists contributed a great deal to meeting the health care needs of the United States. Lillian Wald, the founder of public health nursing in America, operated the Henry Street Settlement primarily through the generosity of a wealthy German-Jewish philanthropist, Jacob Schiff. "Between him and Lillian Wald arose a curious relationship: he helped defray costs on condition that his part be kept secret and she sent him monthly letters detailing her activities"(2). Florence Nightingale had her own well-endowed private purse, which she often used when the bureaucracy of the military establishment tried to block supply requisitions.

It is unrealistic to see Wald and Nightingale as model reformers or agents of change without examining the economic base from which they operated. Today, even with the attendant tax advantages, philanthropists cannot provide for the health needs of America because of the high costs. In addition, there is so much competition for funds that dependence on philanthropy provides shaky economic underpinnings.

System Dilemmas

While the costs of maintaining the system have been rising, the structure of the system has been increasing in complexity. This complexity is emphasized by a quick glance at the organization chart in Table 2-1, which ". . . gives some idea of the many agencies and levels involved in the process of delivering care. The table does not include any of the institutions such as medical, dental, and nursing schools that feed the personnel into the 'system' nor the industries which supply the 'system' "(3). Compounding this complexity is the autonomous functioning of each subsystem that is responsible for only a small portion of society's health care needs. Individual providers who, for the most part, have no formal relationships with each other and who also function autonomously further add to the complexity. Then when providers are added, it becomes an unmanageable labyrinth.

Voluntary collaboration is the major, and some say, the only, connecting thread between the subsystems. It is a weak thread. Incentives for voluntary collaboration among the subsystems have been minimal. Collaboration within the medical subsystem has only occurred because of economic incentives of the referral system. The rise of the medical specialties in the 1930s lessened competition among physicians and fostered economic interdependence and ultimately collaboration. If physicians did not collaborate and cooperate with other physicians, they could be boycotted in the referral system and forced to face financial ruin. Nursing and its subsystems have no such incentives.

It is difficult for nurse providers to define their roles and relationships in this organized complexity. Legally, they must practice nursing within the constraints of the licensure law in their states. Philosophically, they must practice according to their own definition of nursing, often the altruistic, humanistic model. Realistically, nurses must satisfy the needs and demands of the organization, since nurses are usually employees and not private

36

Table 2–1. Spectrum of Health Care Delivery

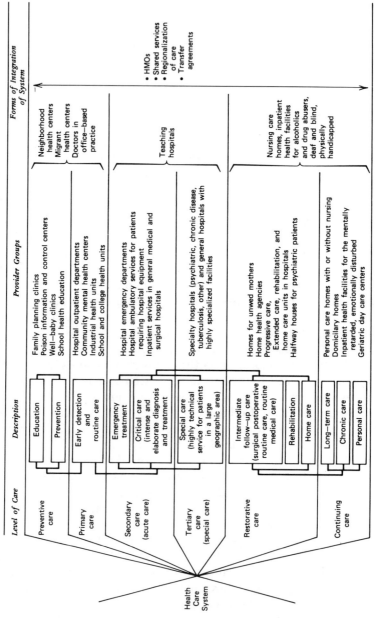

Level of Care	Description	Provider Groups	Forms of Integration of System
Preventive care	Education	Family planning clinics Poison information and control centers Well–baby clinics School health education	Neighborhood health centers Migrant health centers Doctors in office—based practice
	Prevention		
Primary care	Early detection and routine care	Hospital outpatient departments Community mental health centers Industrial health units School and college health units	
Secondary care (acute care)	Emergency treatment	Hospital emergency departments Hospital ambulatory services for patients requiring hospital equipment Inpatient services in general medical and surgical hospitals	Teaching hospitals
	Critical care (intense and elaborate diagnosis and treatment)		
Tertiary care (special care)	Special care (highly technical service for patients in a large geographic area)	Specialty hospitals (psychiatric, chronic disease, tuberculosis, other) and general hospitals with highly specialized facilities	
Restorative care	Intermediate follow–up care (surgical postoperative routine care, routine medical care)	Homes for unwed mothers Home health agencies Progressive care, Extended care, rehabilitation, and home care units in hospitals Halfway houses for psychiatric patients	Nursing care homes, inpatient health facilities for alcoholics and drug abusers, deaf and blind, physically handicapped
	Rehabilitation		
	Home care		
Continuing care	Long–term care	Personal care homes with or without nursing Domiciliary homes Inpatient health facilities for the mentally retarded, emotionally disturbed Geriatric day care centers	
	Chronic care		
	Personal care		

Forms of Integration of System:
- HMOs
- Shared services
- Regionalization of care
- Transfer agreements

Health Care System

Source: HEW, Public Health Service. HRA, Health Planning Information Series, *Trends Affecting U.S. Health Care System,* 1976, p. 262.

business entrepreneurs like physicians. The goals of law, philosophy, and practicality are inevitably in conflict. What are nurses to do? What would you do in the following situation?

The nursing staff on 2 South has asked you, the psychiatric nursing clinical specialist, to consult with them concerning a young patient, Mrs. F., who is having difficulty adjusting to her recent mastectomy. You assess her needs and work with the nursing staff to develop a plan to meet those needs. While you are noting this plan on the patient's chart, the surgeon confronts you. "What are you doing seeing _my_ patient and writing on _my_ chart?" he asks. You explain fully, and he replies, "I am able to meet _my_ patient's needs without your help. I don't want any minipsychiatrist meddling with _my_ patients. You are never to get involved with any of _my_ patients." Despite your attempts to explain, he refuses to talk with you.

Is it ethical to deny a patient a service provided by an organization because one member objects? Is it more important for the organization to function free of conflict than to meet the needs of a patient? Should the physician be the captain of the ship and manage all patient care?

Relationships among health care providers are further complicated by the fact that some functions of medicine are becoming part of nursing. In a certain teaching hospital, the resident physician must take the apical pulse but the nurse gives the intravenous medication. The following anecdote highlights the basic dilemma of the above situation.

A marquis at the court of Louis XV unexpectedly returned from a journey and, on entering his wife's boudoir, found her in the arms of a bishop. After a moment's hesitation, the marquis walked calmly to the window, leaned out, and began going through the motions of blessing the people in the street.

"What are you doing?" cried the anguished wife.

"Monseigneur is performing my functions, so I am performing his"(4).

Clarification of roles may be desirable, but it may not be possible because of rapidly expanding technology and the size and complexity of the system. It seems unlikely that this role ambiguity will disappear in the near future. Ambiguity may be useful in that it creates a situation that forces us to think about how we deal with and relate to others. In addition, it provides time for experimentation before conclusive action has to be taken(5).

The number of health care workers has doubled since the 1950s, and new categories of workers, such as the nurse practitioner and the physician's assistant, are evolving. Although nurse practitioners have been widely accepted by consumers and, in some cases, are preferred over physicians, such acceptance is not universal. A New Jersey nurse practitioner is being sued by the family of a child for whom she prescribed a medication. Although the medication was appropriate and the child suffered no ill effects, the situation is being used as a test case of the scope and role of the nurse practitioner(6). In addition to the confusion and controversy over scope and role of nurse practitioners, there is concern and confusion because they disorder the medical hierarchy.

The nurse practitioner movement was seen initially as a way of providing health care to people who were not otherwise well served. The nurse practitioner movement has evolved in three stages: precursor period (1963 – 1969); role definition and legitimization stage (1970 – 1974); and role consolidation and maturation stage (beginning in 1975)(7). Maturation is incomplete because reimbursement for the services of nurse practitioners from the government and third parties has not been approved. One reason for this is that in some states nurse practitioners cannot practice independently but only along with a physician, because they are required to be under the supervision of a physician. Why is this so? If they are practicing nursing, they may require the support and collaboration of nursing peers but not the supervision of a physician. Some nurse practitioners do function independently but they provide nursing care only. Does this further fragment the care provided by this complex system? Is the move to require practice jointly with a physician an attempt to legitimatize the nurse practitioner or an effort to get around the amorphous boundaries of nursing?

Until recently, the government has called them "physician extenders." Ambiguity over the type and scope of practice of nurse practitioners may be resolved by research aimed at defining the service they provide (is it medicine, nursing, or something else) and by a study of the quality and type of services they provide.

System Evaluation

Evaluation of health services has been piecemeal and uncoordinated. Providers have always been concerned with quality, but standards were not developed until recently. Since 1973 the ANA has published standards for nursing service, nursing practice, nursing education, and continuing nursing education. The movement for evaluation of services has come from outside the provider professions as well. Recent attempts to evaluate quality, such as from the Professional Standards Review Organization (PSRO), were concerned with quality as well as cost containment. Linking federal reimbursement to quality of care was authorized by the Social Security Act of 1972 but nothing of consequence was ever done to implement this portion of the Act. Health services can be evaluated in several ways:

· By structure or quantitative measures, such as the number of hospital beds per population.
· By process, such as what service is provided and how well a person moves through the system.
· By outcomes, such as what happens in terms of cure(1, p. 14).

Each of these measurement techniques has weaknesses. For example, in measuring outcomes, does a death indicate that a patient received poor care? Conversely, if a patient recovers does that mean he or she received good care? What if the patient who recovers was suffering from a cold for which there is no recognized effective treatment? The evaluation process in health care is no less complex than the system itself, and no adequate evaluation tool is now in use.

HEALTH CARE ORGANIZATION

What impact have the American Nurses Association and the American Medical Association had on the evolution of the health care system? In 1950, the ANA endorsed a resolution that the organization itself would not oppose or endorse a national health insurance plan but that individual members should feel free to take either position. In 1958 the organization reaffirmed its position that nursing services should be included as a benefit of any prepaid health insurance plan and at the same time resolved to support extension and improvement of health insurance for beneficiaries of old age, survivors, and disability insurance. Eight years later, in 1966, the ANA resolved to work for the efficient use of nursing personnel, to support the efforts of governmental agencies in the administration of the amendments to the Social Security Act of 1965 (which created Medicare and Medicaid), and to plan for the provision of needed services along with government, community, and professional groups. In 1968 the ANA delegates voted to support comprehensive health planning and urged participation of their membership in such planning. The ANA delegates resolved in 1970 to pressure the government to redefine its priorities in order to put health first, to introduce legislation for a national health insurance plan that would provide for improved use of resources and more incentives for better service, and to contain costs. Although national health insurance was to be the ANA's main objective between 1970 and 1972, little was done because of internal financial difficulties. During this time, nursing representatives testified in Congress on behalf of increased funding and authority for planning agencies, increased consumer participation in the planning of health care, better care for Americans neglected by the health care system, and peer review. In 1974 ANA delegates endorsed resolutions calling for national health insurance, participation in PSRO, nurses as primary care providers, and reimbursement for services of nurses(8).

In contrast, the AMA supported initial efforts toward compulsory health insurance in the early twentieth century but began to oppose any government involvement in health care shortly thereafter. By 1933 the AMA had estabished a firm position against voluntary and compulsory health insurance, which, in effect, was endorsing the status quo. There was some dissension in medical circles, but the AMA held firmly to its position and prevailed. The amendments to the Social Security Act of 1965, which established Medicare and Medicaid, had been proposed by Presidents Roosevelt, Truman, and Kennedy but were vigorously opposed by the AMA. Although the AMA supported the Hill-Burton Act, in general it has a record of opposing government involvement in medical care, health insurance, physician training, and direct support of medical schools—all of which have taken place in recent years. The AMA also opposed the Professional Standards Review Organization (PSRO) but agreed to assist in its implementation after its creation in 1972.

In retrospect, the ANA has had a liberal, populist record on external issues, while the AMA has adopted a conservative posture on the same issues. In recent years, the ANA has been more politically astute than the AMA in assuming a consumer advocate position and in seeing, if not welcoming, the inevitability of government involvement in health care. The differences in viewpoint between the ANA and the AMA may be due in part to the constituencies of the two organizations. Nurses tended to come from less affluent backgrounds and to have lower incomes than physicians, which may partially explain the tendency of nurses to adopt more populist attitudes. On internal issues, the ANA has been conservative, not wishing to offend any of its large and diverse constituency.

The ANA, formed in 1896, is the official voice of nursing, although it represents only approximately 20% of all registered nurses. To place this figure in perspective, it is helpful to know that the AMA represents approximately 60% of all licensed physicians. Joanne Ashley explains the political ramifications of these numbers:

> From the beginning, the nurses associations were a minority group among nurses. . . . Fearing failure because their group constituted a minority and in order to avoid antagonism and division. . . members agreed early that assuming a conciliatory attitude was best(9).

The ANA has always been at a disadvantage because of the diversity of its constituency. The AMA seems to have less of a problem in this area than the ANA. When physicians graduate from their basic program, they have all been through essentially the same learning experiences and are considered equal. This is not the case in nursing, and the ANA often is blamed for failing to represent nursing when there is little agreement on what nursing is.

The National League for Nursing (NLN) was formed in 1952 through the consolidation of six nursing organizations. Membership is open to any person or agency interested in nursing, whereas the ANA admits only nurses to membership. The NLN, with approximately 17,000 individual members and 1,800 agency members, and the ANA have some overlap in their functions and purpose (see Table 2-2). In its functions the NLN lists working with the ANA to advance nursing. Notably absent from the ANA's list of functions is any mention of the NLN. Although the NLN has focused on evaluation and accreditation of educational programs, and the ANA has focused on standards of practice, education, and welfare of nurses, territorial skirmishes between the two organizations are inevitable. Competition is valuable in open systems, but is the competition between these two organizations important or is it detrimental to nursing?

Some members have criticized the nursing organizations for failing to meet their clinical needs. In 1968 a group of cardiac nurses approached the ANA to explore the possibilities of creating a specialty subsystem within the ANA but were rejected because the ANA felt it was not prepared structurally for a specialty group. These nurses organized the American Association of Cardiovascular Nurses (the name was changed to the American Association of Critical Care Nurses in 1971). Its purpose was "to provide cardiovascular nurses of the nation a representative association that would promote the exchange of scientific knowledge in the field of cardiovascular nursing"(10). Two years after its formation, the association had 500 members. Two years later, in 1972, it had 9,600 members. The association's growth rate has continued to be dramatic, and current membership is over 33,000 nurses. Has the ANA failed to meet the needs of nurses?

The ANA published its first code of ethics in 1926. This code recognized the nurse as the coworker of the physician with a relationship of mutual respect and favored continuing education and legislative involvement of nurses. Ethical issues of concern to ANA members were, however, more mundane that year: uniform requirements, participation of nurses in commercial advertising, nurses functioning as anesthetists, nurses working in the offices of chiropractors or osteopaths, and nurses outlining diabetic diets in the absence of the attending physician.

The importance of legislative involvement was not new to nursing. In 1908 Dock chided members of the Nurses Associated Alumnae, the precursor of the ANA, for failing to support a resolution supporting women's right to vote:

Dear Editor: Since the historic meeting in September, 1896, in the Manhattan Beach Hotel when you and a little group of women, who were very loyal to their profession and the cause of women generally, met, to bring the Nurses' Associated Alumnae into being, I have never been disappointed in the actions of that body, of which you and I are charter members, until this year, when I read, with humiliation, I must frankly say, that a negative vote "by a large majority" was recorded at San Francisco against the reasonable and temperately expressed suffrage resolution offered to it!

It was a shock, because, though I know many nurses have never given the subject a thought, yet I believed that they might always be depended upon, in their associations, to take instinctively the intelligent and above all the sympathetic position on large human questions. I am far from thinking that nurses have time or strength for work outside of their own field, and do not expect to see them actively engaged in the equality movement, but to give moral support and endorsement takes no time; to feel intelligent sympathy costs no money.

There are no reasons against political equality for women except selfish ones, and every good reason for it. May I run over a few of them? First, the patriotic reason: to deny the sacred duty of citizenship is to deny the foundation principle on which our democracy is built. As for the practical common sense reasons, they are on every hand. To help bring about more just and equal opportunities and equal pay for self-supporting women; to aid in the great child-saving crusade against the horrors of child labor; to carry good home-making and sanitary housekeeping into our city governments—why, I could not count all the reasons, but let me come down to concrete instances. A couple of years ago the Associated Alumnae passed a resolution endorsing the Pure Food law. That was quite right, but now they reject a woman-suffrage resolution, although, if the housekeepers of the nation had votes, we could have had a Pure Food law twenty years ago.

Next, our state societies have all responded warmly to Mrs. Crane's almshouse propaganda. Again good, but look here? what's the matter with our almshouses? Men's con-

Table 2-2. Comparison of ANA and NLN

	ANA	NLN
Year formed	1897	1952[a]
Membership	Individual RNs only	Individual nurses, health care providers, and other interested individuals and agencies
Number of members	Approximately 181,000[b]	Approximately 17,000 individuals and 1,800 agencies [c]
Purpose	To foster high standards of nursing practice, to promote the professional and educational advancement of nurses, and to promote the welfare of nurses to the end that all people may have better nursing care[d]	To foster the development and improvement of hospital, industrial, public health, and other organized nursing services and of nursing education through the coordinated action of nurses, allied professional groups, citizens, agencies, and schools to the end that the nursing needs of the people will be met[e]
Functions	1. To establish functions, standards, and qualifications for nursing practice 2. To enunciate standards of nursing education and implement them through appropriate channels 3. To enunciate standards of nursing service and implement them through appropriate channels 4. To establish a code of ethical conduct for practicioners 5. To stimulate and promote research designed to enlarge the knowledge on which the practice of nursing is based	1. To identify the nursing needs of society and to foster programs designed to meet these needs 2. To develop and support services for the improvement of nursing care and nursing education through consultation, testing, accreditation, evaluation, and other activities 3. To work with the American Nurses Association for the advancement of nursing 4. To work with voluntary, government, and other agencies and groups toward the achievement of comprehensive health care 5. To respond in appropriate ways to universal nursing needs

6. To promote legislation and to speak for nurses in regard to legislative action

7. To promote and protect the economic and general welfare of nurses

8. To provide professional record service and assist states with counseling and placement activities

9. To provide for the continuing professional development of practitioners

10. To represent nurses and serve as their spokesperson with allied national and international organizations, government bodies, and the public

11. To serve as the official representative of the nurses in the United States as a member of the International Council of Nurses

12. To promote the general health and welfare of the public through all association programs, relationships, and activities

13. To promote relationships with the National Student Nurses Association

---

[a] Six organizations, the oldest of which was formed in 1893, merged to form NLN. These organizations included the National League of Nursing Education, the National Organization of Public Health Nursing, Association of Collegiate Schools of Nursing, National Association of Colored Graduate Nurses, American Association of Industrial Nurses.

[b] American Nurses Association, December, 1979.

[c] National League for Nursing, December, 1979.

[d] Bylaws, American Nurses Association, 1978.

[e] Bylaws, National League for Nursing, 1979.

trol everywhere and no women with any authority to see that they are managed humanely. If women had votes, even municipal ones, as they have in England, we might get women on as overseers of the poor, where they ought to be. I have just had very interesting light on a large almshouse, where an excellent woman is matron. She has no authority at all, and told a lady of my acquaintance that she and the physician appealed over and over again to the county supervisors for *necessary* comforts and improvements for the poor and the sick, "but," she says, "they are not interested; they do not care, and they do not listen." How foolish for us to take up an almshouse propaganda and yet reject the belief that women should vote!

Again, our nurses are becoming keenly interested in the tuberculosis propaganda, and this is well and right. But of all things in the world the tuberculosis question is a social question and the causes of tuberculosis (outside of the bacillus) are social causes which need the ballot for their changing, such as bad housing, overwork, underpay, neglect of childhood, etc. Take the present question of underfed school children in New York. How many of them will have tuberculosis? If mothers and nurses had votes there might be school lunches for all those children and, as often suggested, teaching could accompany the cooking and serving.

I hope that at a future meeting our members will reconsider their hasty snapshot verdict(11).

Reprinted with permission of the American Nurses Association. See reference 13.

KOAN

Dock's position was clear: nursing organizations should be involved in social issues of the time. What should be the role of nursing organizations on issues peripheral to the purpose of the system? What is a peripheral issue?

In 1946, the ANA adopted an economic security program for nurses that included collective bargaining because previous attempts to improve the working conditions of nurses had been ineffective. Ashley feels that the lack of success was due to the fact that nurses underestimated the strength of their opposition. Physicians and hospital administrators worked together to keep nurses in their place. Kalisch and Kalisch agree that the nurses' collective bargaining movement resulted from nurses' attempts, which were thwarted by physicians, to increase their responsibility(12). Although the American work force has grown in numbers, the percentage of union members has declined except in the health care system. The number of nurses in collective bargaining units is increasing, with the ANA being the major collective bargaining agent for nurses. The American Hospital Association opposes this move by nurses to gain power through collective bargaining on the grounds that the resulting fragmentation of responsibility violates principles of sound management.

The ANA's role as a collective bargaining agent has been questioned by members who are in management positions and are placed in an adversary (however friendly) role during negotiations. A recent labor relations board decision agreed that the Maryland Nurses Association was not an appropriate collective bargaining agent because its board of directors included nurses in hospital management positions. The implications of this decision, certain to be challenged in higher courts, are important. If the decision is upheld, the ANA will have to make a choice between being a professional organization and being a collective bargaining agent. Associations in two states have already made this decision and have withdrawn from their collective bargaining programs(13).

Collective bargaining, which is essentially a rule-making process, was foreseen as a major factor for change in the health care industry. However, conclusive research is not available to show whether nursing care or job satisfaction among nurses is better in labor-organized hospitals. Perhaps too much hope had been placed in the collective bargaining process as the answer to the problem of oppression of nurses. This is not to deny the effectiveness of collective action by nurses, but a clear understanding of all the forces of change discussed throughout other chapters of this text is needed.

SYSTEM IMBALANCES

A lack of balance among subsystems has accentuated the weaknesses of the health care and nursing systems. Tension among subsystems in any system helps to keep the system balanced and functioning. A current problem is the balance in nursing between individuation and integration into the larger system. Nurses are displaying their individuation through participation in self-assertiveness movements, through support of licensure laws that reflect nurses' accountability as well as differences between medicine and nursing, and through independent practice activity. Integration, or incorporation through teamwork into the larger system, which is the balance of individuation, is equally valuable for a system's functioning.

KOAN

For several months public health nurse M. has been providing agency supplies to a poor client who is unable to obtain them through any other means. This is contrary to agency policy. The nurse is following the altruistic model in a system that subscribes to the economic model. She is displaying self-assertiveness rather than integration. What should she do? How would you solve this dilemma?

Another imbalance currently receiving attention is the emphasis on medical technology representing the yang of Eastern philosophy, or the Western ideal of curing, as opposed to the yin, or humanistic, caring elements of health care. The latter, which had been devalued, are experiencing a resurgence of interest in the holistic health care movement. This imbalance is illustrated by Czoniczer:

> Technologized medicine has created the ambivalent patient who, *as an object of medical treatment,* is better off than ever before: the cause of his illness can be traced with

greater speed and precision than at any other time; his chances for recovery, rehabilitation and a lengthened life are better than at any other former period in history. On the other hand, his position *as a suffering anxiety-filled human being* is not enviable: the *Ars Medici;* the human component, an integral part of medicine, far from keeping pace with technical innovations, seems to be vanishing. There is now an immense gap between medicine's scientific and its human performances, and that is why today the illness-ridden, suffering human being does not fare as well as should be expected in the "Golden Age of Medicine"(14).

In addition to the yin-yang imbalance in the services provided, there is an imbalance in the patient-provider relationship. The patient has become too passive and the provider too powerful. A sharing of power, a balance, is needed. Czoniczer believes people walk into a physician's office expecting too much, because profit-oriented technological companies have used media to make Americans illness and quick-cure oriented. People have been taught to expect instant cure through medication for many stress-related health problems that they themselves could control without medication(14, p.19).

A dynamic balance among shareholders, providers, and patients in the health care system is not evident. The imbalance of power between physician and patient is compounded by the disparity of power between providers. Physician providers, though fewer in number than nurse providers, have much more power. A dynamic balance occurs when each corner of the triangle in Figure 2-1 has an equal amount of power. Tension between the subsystems keeps the system in balance and facilitates functioning.

Managing the complex health care system, which has been out of balance for a long period of time, is a challenge. It has been said

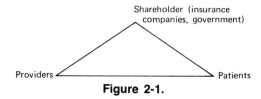

Figure 2-1.

that health care institutions have not met this challenge. Drucker sees several alibis being used to excuse the ineffectiveness of service institutions: the managers are not businesslike, the institutions need better people, the objectives and results of service institutions are intangible. Drucker believes that because service institutions serve large constituencies they try to please everyone, which results in a lack of concentration, and that better management will be forthcoming when service institutions clearly define their objectives, set their priorities, and evaluate their results(15).

In complex organizations it is difficult for managers to achieve their ends only through the use of persuasion and formal authority. Successful managers use a variety of techniques and change their style to fit different situations. Managers attempt to create order in an organization, while leaders create disorder. There are many other differences between managers and leaders; these differences are detailed in Table 2-3(16).

Nurses in management positions, such as directors of nursing, are often expected to be both managers and leaders. In a hospital, for example, the director of nursing is given the task of managing the largest subsystem in the organization but is frequently not given the support either from within the nursing system or from the larger system. Few people, if any, can be both manager and leader. What is it that we expect from nurses in management positions? Where are nursing's leaders?

KOAN

Organization issues identified by four nursing leaders are contained in Table 2-4(20). What other issues related to the organization of the health care system or the nursing system can you identify?

The director of nursing, usually a female functioning in a male-dominated system, experiences additional stresses because of her sex. The female executive must constantly fight stereotypes, training, and conditioning. In a study of solitary women in a small professional peer group, Frank found that the woman is

Table 2–3. Differences Between Managers and Leaders [a]

	Manager	Leader
Definition	Attempts to solve problems	Attempts to direct affairs
Needed traits	Persistence, toughmindedness, hard work, intelligence, analytical ability, tolerance, good will, instinct for survival, ability to tolerate mundane	Likes to seek out risk and danger when reward and opportunity appear high
Creates	Order	Disorder
Attitudes toward goals	Impersonal, if not passive; goals arise out of necessity rather than out of desires and therefore are deeply imbedded in the history and culture of the organization	Personal and active; influence exerted by a leader in altering moods, evoking images and expectations, and establishing specific desires and objectives determines direction a business will take
Conceptions of work	An enabling process involving some combination of people and ideas interacting to establish strategies and make decisions	Work is to develop fresh approaches to long-standing problems and to open issues for new options; ideas occupy, at times, obsess the leader's mental life
Techniques	Range of methods including calculating the interests of the opposition, staging and timing the surfacing of controversial issues, reducing tensions, negotiating and bargaining, using rewards and punishments, coordinating and balancing continually, acting to limit choices	Is an integral part of the product, projecting ideas into images that excite people and then developing choices that give the projected images substance; works from high risk positions

Table 2–3. (Continued)

	Manager	Leader
Aim	Shifting balance of power toward solutions acceptable as a compromise among conflicting values, reconciling differences, converting win-lose situations to win-win situations	Creating excitement in work; profoundly altering human, economic, and political relationships
Described by subordinates	Inscrutable, detached, manipulative; purpose is to maintain controlled, rational, and equitable structure	Descriptions are rich in emotional content—attracts strong feelings of identification, love, or hate
Relations with others	Prefers to work with people, avoids solitary activity because it creates anxiety, seeks others out to work with, collaborates, maintains low level of emotional involvement in working relationships, may not intuitively sense the thoughts and feelings of others (may not have empathy capacity to take in emotional signals and make them mean something in a relationship with another person), relates to people according to the role they play in a sequence of events or in a decision-making process, concerned with roles in the process and how to get things done, communicates indirectly using signals instead of messages because the signal is less clear, plays for time so that compromises will emerge that take the sting out of win-lose situations	Concerned with ideas in a more intuitive and empathetic way, concerned with what events and decisions mean to participants, involved in relationships that are turbulent, intense, at times disorganized

Impacts on organization	Focuses on decision-making process, interest in tactics makes organization fatter in bureaucratic and political intrigue and leaner in direct, hard activity and warm human relations	Intensifies individual motivation and often produces unanticipated results
Sense of self	In harmony with environment, conservator and regulator of an existing order with which has personal identity and from which gains rewards, sense of self-worth enhanced by working to perpetuate and strengthen existing institutions, harmonizes with ideals of duty and responsibility, self-esteem grows through participation and conformity	Sense of profound separateness from environment including other people, may work in an organization but never belongs to it, sense of self does not depend on memberships, work roles, or other social indicators of identity
Background	Life has been more or less peaceful	Life marked by continual struggle to attain some sense of order

[a] Adopted with permission from Zalesnik A: Managers and leaders: are they different? *Harvard Business Review*, 55(3):67–69, 1977. Vol. 55, No. 3, pps. 67–79.

Table 2–4. Organizational Issues in Nursing [a]

Well, I think one of the issues in nursing—not precisely in education—is, what is the American Nurses Association (ANA) doing and going to do. I have some qualms about the emphasis upon collective bargaining and the economics side of it. I feel very strongly about the strikes. . . . I think the Commission on Education has been absolutely dormant until very recently. . . . I think they should have taken a very much more active role than they have. . . . I think what the ANA has done about the Position Paper is incredible. I think their statement in 1973 relative to diploma programs was unbelievable, *unbelievable!* The ANA has done nothing since 1965 but dilute the Position Paper, which has been the official position of the association since 1965. Another issue might be which organization should be responsible for accreditation of nursing programs. I happen to believe that accreditation belongs in the ANA or under its general auspices. I do not believe it belongs in a nonnursing organization.

Mildred Montag (p. 228)

I think the biggest issue is how much unanimity of purpose we can hope for in a profession as diverse as our own. Internal warfare in the nursing profession is scandalous. Antagonism between the ANA and the National League for Nursing (NLN) is a case in point. Another is continuing mutual criticism of nursing education and nursing service. A more recent one is the emerging chasm between nursing administrators and nursing staff, precipitated by Taft-Hartley revisions.

Mary Kelly Mullane (p. 252)

Picking out any one thing, of course, is really never that simple; but if I were going to identify one single thing, then I would say differentiation of professional and technical careers in nursing, legally and openly and honestly, is the most critical point that we have because all of these other things will fall into shape, once careers are openly admitted and lead to honest recruitment, for example. We would begin to be honest and accountable to the public, which we

Table 2−4. *(Continued)*

are not. We would quit the head-in-sand cover-up. We would begin to develop a little self-respect. We are so busy apologizing to hospital school graduates that it gets to be pretty bad. I wonder when we are going to start apologizing for what we are doing to baccalaureate graduates. The human waste in terms of knowledge; the misuse of graduates; the human waste in students; and the financial cost to parents who invest money in their children to send them to college and then have them leave nursing because what happens in the real world is "for the birds." What about the public, who are denied not only any guarantee of professional services, but even their existence?

Martha Rogers (p. 328)

I would say this, that to me patients, sick people, are not getting good care. I believe in prevention; I think a lot of things could happen in the community in the way of prevention. I think there will always be sick people, and, to me, if one gets good care in the hospital today, it's accidental rather than planned. This saddens me. Of course this was what my whole life work has been about. The forces that operate against good nursing care are tremendously strong, and they include not only hospital administrators and doctors; they include a tremendous number of nurses, who really don't want to change things.

Dorothy Smith (p. 381)

[a] Table and all quotations taken, with permission, from reference 17.

labeled as a bitch, a bird, or a babe and ostracized as an intruder. When the woman tried to influence the group, she was ignored and accepted defeat without a fight(18).

The nurse managers face a most difficult task: the system is out of balance, expectations of them from both inside and outside the nursing system are unrealistic, and little support is available. What can be done? Collective bargaining and self-assertiveness of nurses have created some change, but there is much more to do in the effort to restore balance and to create a more efficient health care system. Nurse managers need to develop and refine their management skills and to focus on working *for* the nurses they manage. Nurses need to support each other and their managers. The nursing system needs to devote more time and energy to development of risk-taking nurse leaders. External forces that are pressing for the attainment of a balanced, efficient system must be exploited. Are we prepared for these challenges? These and other challenges will be discussed in following chapters.

REFERENCES

1. Judd LR, McEwen RJ: *A Handbook for Consumer Participation in Health Care Planning.* Chicago, Blue Cross Association, 1977, pp 3–4.

2. Howe I: *World of Our Fathers.* New York, Simon & Schuster Inc, 1976, p 91.

3. *Trends Affecting U.S. Health Care System,* US Department of Health, Education and Welfare, 1976, p 262.

4. Koestler A: *Janus: A Summing Up.* New York, Random House Inc, 1978, p 112.

5. Pascale RT: Zen and the art of management. *Harvard Business Review* 56:155 March–April 1978.

6. Nurse practitioners fight moves to restrict their practice. *Am J Nurs* 78:1285, 1308, August 1978.

7. Edmunds M: Evaluation of nurse practitioner effectiveness: An overview of the literature. *Evaluation and the Health Professions* 1:42–47, Spring 1978.

8. Flanagan Lyndia: *One Strong Voice: The Story of the American Nurses Association.* Kansas City, Missouri, 1976.

9. Ashley J: *Hospitals, Paternalism and the Role of the Nurse.* New York, Teachers College Press, 1977, p 98.

10. *Bylaws.* The American Association of Critical Care Nurses 1978.

11. Dock L: The suffrage question. *Am J Nurs* 8:925–927, August, 1908.

12. Kalisch BJ, Kalisch PA: An analysis of the sources of physician-nurse conflict. *J Nurs Adm* 8:51–57, January 1977.

13. State association drops union status to win support for new practice act. *RN* 42:12, 1979.

14. Czoniczer G: The role of the patient in modern medicine, *Man and Medicine* 3:17, 1978.

15. Drucker, PF: *Management: Tasks, Responsibilities, Practices.* New York, Harper & Row Publishers Inc, 1974, p 137.

16. Zaleznik A: Managers and leaders: Are they different? *Harvard Business Review* 55:67–79, 1977.

17. Safier G: *Contemporary American Leaders in Nusring: An Oral History.* New York, McGraw Hill & Company Inc, 1977, pp 228, 252, 328, 381.

18. Frank H: *Women in the Organization.* Philadelphia, University of Pennsylvania Press, 1977, p 37.

CHAPTER THREE

Power, Conflict, Collaboration

Power is the ability to cause or prevent change. It has two dimensions. One is power as potentiality, or latent power. This is power that has not yet been fully developed; it is the ability to cause a change at some future time. We speak of this future change as *possibility*, a word which comes directly from the same root as power, namely *posse*, to be able. The other dimension is power as actuality.

*R. May**

POWER, VALUES, AND LEADERSHIP

Only in the past several years has the use of power been an openly discussed issue for nurses. Nursing of late, has been preoccupied with the issue of power as evidenced by recent literature and workshop or convention topics. According to McClelland, power orientation and development can be grouped into four categories or stages[2]:

1. Object of power: Self; to feel stronger
   Source of power: External phenomena (God, mother, leader, food) strengthen me

*From reference 1.

2. Object of power: Self; to strengthen, control, direct self
   Source of power: Self; internal phenomena (autonomy, willpower) strengthen me
3. Object of power: Others; to influence
   Source of power: Self; internal phenomena (assertiveness, desire to experience power) strengthen me
4. Object of power: Others; to serve or influence others
   Source of power: External phenomena (religion, law, group values) strengthen me

People in the first stage of power development prefer to talk, to share, and to nurture. As people move to stage two, they place emphasis on outward control of expressions of anger and on attempts to be independent. Characteristic of the second stage are a feeling of disillusionment with scientific knowledge and a desire for knowledge of how to control things better. When people move to the third stage, they are concerned with prestige and possessions. In this stage the goal is power rather than achievement. By stage four, the final stage, people have developed loyalty to a higher authority, and they view their power-related actions in terms of duty or responsibility to a higher authority.

When power orientation is viewed developmentally, each category or stage includes a crisis to be resolved before preceding to the next stage. According to Erikson's theory of human development*, each crisis is resolved by striking a balance between extremes but reoccurs in some form at other points during development. Maturation into stage four is evidenced by showing concern for group values, translating those values into goals, taking the initiative in formulating means to accomplish the goals, and instilling in members of the group a sense of confidence in their ability to achieve the goals.

Authority figures can be found at all four levels of power orientation. However, according to McClelland, to be effective leaders in any stage must make their followers feel powerful, strong, and capable(2, p. 260). Also, McClelland explains, "people who feel that they are pawns tend to be passive and useless to the leader who gets his satisfaction from dominating them. Slaves are the most inefficient form of labor ever devised by man"(2, p. 263).

---

*Erikson E: *Childhood and Society,* ed 2. New York, WW Norton & Co, 1963.

KOAN

After reviewing McClelland's four stages of power orientation at the beginning of this chapter, where would you place the nursing system? Why have you placed it in that stage? What is the system's source of power?

Over time, unless there is a system of controls, leaders and their followers may begin to believe that the leader and not the group is the source of power. Safeguards against abuses of leadership have been built into the democratic system, for example, through a series of checks and balances. In the United States, for example, there are three branches of government: executive, legislative, and judicial. Each keeps watch over the others, while the public, with its advocacy groups, keeps watch over all three, always alert to abuses of power. "A Martian observer might conclude that as a nation we are excessively, almost obsessively worried about the abuse of power"(2, p. 266).

KOAN

If power is the ability to cause and innocence is the inability to cause or prevent change, and power and innocence are at opposite ends of a continuum, where would you place nursing in that continuum of power?

Since most nurses work in hospitals, it is interesting to examine the system of checks and balances characteristic of a democracy as it operates in a hospital setting. Even though hospitals are patterned on the corporate, hierarchical model rather than on the democratic model, it is useful to survey hospitals for the system of checks and balances they employ to prevent abuses of power. The executive branch is represented by the hospital administrative hierarchy. What group represents the legislative branch? That is, who makes the rules by which the system operates? Most nurses would agree that physicians represent the legislative branch, although the government and third-party insurers are becoming increasingly involved in this process. What then represents the judicial branch—what subsystem enforces the rules and administers justice? Some subsystems of some health care systems rely on collective bargaining agreements to serve the judicial function. In systems where this resource is not available, what recourse does a wronged party have? Consider this situation:

Nurse S. planned to quit her job and move from the area. The hospital policy manual stated that two weeks' notice was required before leaving. She gave her employer three weeks' notice and requested that she be paid her four remaining vacation days. During her last week of work, the personnel director informed her that the hospital was understaffed and that since the hospital preferred four weeks' notice, he would not authorize payment for her four remaining vacation days unless she agreed to work an additional week after her scheduled termination date. Frustrated by attempts to have this decision reversed within the system's hierarchy, she consulted an attorney who advised her that she had a very good case but that winning it would require a considerable investment of time, energy, and money. She returned to the hospital and worked the additional week.

People in large systems have little power when standing alone. Once they decide to work within such a system, they automatically limit their options. Margaret Sanger and Lillian Wald, two important nurse reformers, chose to leave the existing health care system in order to maximize their impact and to achieve their goals. Whether individuals in a system are leaders or followers, their goals will rarely be achieved without the support of others who share the same goals. Attempts by nursing service administrators to implement new nursing delivery systems such as primary care nursing illustrate the problems encountered when members of the group do not back the leaders. For example, nursing administrators who believed that they had solid support for changing a delivery system may find staff nurses reverting to previous patterns. This resistance to major change is common and usually not malicious. Implementation of the change may have lacked adequate planning, including educating the participants, or adequate rewards for the participants. Or staff nurses may not have understood or shared the leader's goal. People who attempt to initiate second-order changes, such as reformation of the established power structures, value systems, relationships, or ways of doing things, begin with a balance between a sense of affiliation and a power motivation, which evolves into an imbalance with the power motivation becoming most important—an "imperial frame of mind"(2, p. 355).

Another factor to assess when this type of problem arises is whether the goals were overshadowed by the process of change itself. American business leaders are examining Japanese techniques for change, where the "grass roots" participate in the problem-solving process with subtle guidance from their leaders. As a result of these techniques, the grass-roots solution is often the solution that management wants, and implementation becomes much easier because the grass roots feel that they participated in the final decision.

The support system for nurses' reform attempts has expanded, and the power value espoused by some nursing leaders is beginning to be recognized as desirable by more nurses. Nurses, in their attempts to gain power, have precipitated what one major newspaper headlined on page 1 as "Nurses and Doctors at War Here and Across the Country," (*Philadelphia Inquirer*, February 2, 1975). Does this mean that war is inevitable? If so, in what subsystem(s) of the health care system will it occur—economic, political, social, or some other subsystem?

KOAN

In the 1960s, reformers struggled to help oppressed blacks by calling for increased black political clout, growth in black pride, and more black capitalism and by nurturing black leaders. Some political observers are now beginning to say that this reform movement has not been as successful as was hoped and that a black backlash may occur. Viewing it from an historical perspective, is this a pattern in American culture? If so, what changes or problems can you predict will result from nursing's attempts to gain power to reform the system?

Social systems are intricately intertwined with political systems. In the hospital, for example, the established, powerful physicians and the members of the board of trustees have many characteristics in common. Their wives often serve on the same community activity committees, they belong to the same country clubs, they attend the same social functions, their children mingle in school, and they buy and service their automobiles at the same place. In the American system of socioeconomic classes, board members and physicians are often equal and often have social alliances outside the hospital. Because of this, physicians' concerns related to the hospital may be given precedence over nurses' concerns. When there is a conflict between physicians and nurses, board members would probably side with the physicians because of their comfortable relationship. Furthermore, physicians have more opportunity to lobby for their position in social settings, and since they are likely to continue as social acquaintances of the board members, the physicians' views are most often supported. One rationale given for this is that the physicians control the "purse strings" of the hospital because they admit patients.

In health care systems run by religious orders, the heirarchical structure within the health care system is often reversed outside of that system. For example, a nun who is the director of nursing reports to a nun who is the hospital administrator, but when they return to the convent, the director of nursing may be the superior of the nun who is the hospital administrator. The role changes required when they enter the door of either system can be very difficult to adjust to.

Power in organizations is not always held by those who appear to have it. Although people in line positions have the authority to make decisions, the people in staff positions may actually make them. A busy legislator's staff, for example, may make decisions after collecting information and formulating a position paper, although the legislator casts the vote. In industry, a frequent caricature is the unhappy and disappointed executive who has been "kicked upstairs" and given an important-sounding title but little responsibility or real power.

Physicians have a unique kind of power—the kind that overrides all other authority under most circumstances. This type of power is termed *Aesculapian authority** and has three compo-

---

*Aesculapius personified Greek medicine. He was first regarded as a perfect physician and later as the god of health. His cult persisted longer than that of any other Greek gods, and it was progressively integrated into Christian tradition.

nents: *(1)* the right to be heard because of the physician's knowledge; *(2)* the right to direct others because of the physician's moral commitment to humanity; and *(3)* the right to direct others because of the physician's mystical association with God. Using this authority, physicians can compel patients to accept directives that they wouldn't accept under other circumstances. Physicians can also exempt patients from normal responsibilities because of illness. "The doctor's authority must carry more weight than all other authorities to which the patient is subject or the doctor cannot perform the function of restricting the patient's activities for the benefit of his health"(3). Aesculapian authority is conferred gradually by colleagues and patients at an earlier age than other types of authority; a medical student is referred to as "doctor." Military or political authority is usually achieved later in life.

Corea details what she considers to be abuses of physicians' power in her book, *The Hidden Malpractice*(4). She cites examples that range from the slowness of *Journal of the American Medical Association* in printing articles critical of birth control pills out of the desire not to offend some of its major advertisers to physicians refusing to treat women on welfare unless these women agree to be sterilized. Corea asks, "Why do doctors prescribe more mood-altering drugs for women than for men? One answer given is that the doctor misinterprets his female patient's symptoms as imaginary because she speaks in a cultural language that he does not understand"(4, p. 83). In addition, it might be said that because of his authority, the doctor doesn't feel that it is necessary to learn the culture and language of oppressed groups. He is allowed to remain unknowing because of his powers, his time constraints, and the wide variety of clientele that he serves. In addition, he is often educated to believe that he has control over nursing decisions.

KOAN

What are your values about power? Which of the following statements do you agree with? Disagree with?

1. **People with power must be watched for abuses of power.**

2. Absolute power corrupts, and power corrupts absolutely.
3. He who appeases the alligator is eaten last.
4. Having power is a comfortable feeling.
5. It is best not to challenge people with power by "making waves."

USES OF POWER

In the 1978 elections, the AMA spent about $1.5 million in supporting candidates (*Philadelphia Inquirer,* November 12, 1978, p. 8). Nursing's special-interest lobby is not nearly as well established or as well funded. In the 1978 elections, the Nurses Coalition for Action in Politics (N-CAP), which is the political action arm of the ANA, had a total of $85,000 to distribute to candidates(5). N-CAP has two functions: *(1)* political education of nurses and, *(2)* endorsements and of contributions to "health-minded individuals who are running for Congress"(6). Thirty-one state nurses associations have political action committees that serve similar functions at the state level. Although nursing organizations will probably never have enough money to pour $1.5 million a year into political campaigns, nurses can have an impact on elections through voting, through volunteering to work for candidates, through working to correct what they feel is wrong on the political scene, through seeking elected or appointed office, or through serving as party convention delegates(6, p. 11–14). Nurses, the largest group of health care providers, have great potential for political impact by virtue of their numbers. Unfortunately this potential has never been fully exploited.

On a smaller scale, nurses holding power can use that power to prepare other nurses for leadership through a mentor relationship. Reflecting on the importance of the mentor relationship, an executive describes the philosophy he found in the organization he joined four decades ago:

[The philosophy was] simply that executive responsibility involves assisting the people down the line to be successful. The boss in any department is the first assistant to those who report to him. You've got to live your life in a worthwhile way. This is a worthwhile philosophy. It doesn't hurt people, it helps them; and after it helps them, it helps the business.

But it was unique for the time. People weren't used to thinking in terms of an upside-down organization in those days. The typical executive was more like a king, saying, "I make all the decisions, and all you little gnomes do my bidding, or else"(7).

Few organizations have a formal mentor program, and not all mentors are found within the organization where a person works. Nightingale and other early leaders including Nutting and Stewart developed close relationships with people within the existing political and health-power structures of the day and used those relationships to accomplish their goals. Some early leaders also developed close, helping relationships with their peers in nursing, which increased their strength as leaders. In a recent lament, one prominent nurse said:

What has happened to the art of mentorship? Why don't senior nurses reach out to help young staff who are so obviously in need of strong support? And, conversely, why don't young nurses seek that counsel instead of isolating themselves in a web of anxiety. When the young don't seek and the mature don't offer, both are deprived(8).

Power in the Caring Relationship

Each care giver and receiver brings to the helping relationship personal motives and self-concepts. The motives include affiliation (to be accepted), power, and achievement. Power must be shared by both the care giver and the receiver, and the task to be accomplished must be agreed upon by both. Tasks range from tieing a shoe to improving organizational effectiveness. If, for example, the giver wants the receiver to switch from a homosexual to a heterosexual life-style, to stop smoking, or to lose weight, and the receiver does not choose to change, none of these goals will be accomplished. All goals must be shared by care giver and receiver for change to occur.

The environment in which the helping occurs is important to the relationship. If one of the three motives (power, affiliation, achievement) is excessively rewarded, it can affect the entire relationship. In the learning environment, for example, if student achievement becomes the primary motive, the student will experience intense peer competition and will probably not learn the value of using peers as a resource for support and learning. If faculty control over students is the primary motive, an adversary relationship between teacher and learner will evolve. With this in mind, directors of progressive nursing programs have appointed students to decision-making committees to facilitate the sharing of power and have encouraged affiliation through seminars and informal gatherings to promote the exchange of ideas and feelings.

In the nurse-client relationship, "nurses tend to rely upon unicultural professional values which are largely derived from our dominant Anglo-American caring values and behavioral expectations" according to Leninger, who feels a change is needed(9). Leninger also says:

> Nursing theory and practice must take into account man's cultural and social behavior so that the nurse's mode of thinking and interacting with individuals will reflect new and penetrating views about behavior in health and illness. Understanding the culture of an individual seeking health care is just as important for effective health care as is knowledge of the physiological and psychological aspects of an individual's illness"(9, p. 110).

Knowledge of the patient's ethnicity will equip the helper with an understanding of the receiver's motives, self-concept, and view of the task to be accomplished.

The power motive in the helping relationship is a difficult concept for nurses to accept. In their book, *Politics of Pain Management: Staff-Patient Interaction,* Fagerhaugh and Strauss examine power in pain management.

> As we shall repeatedly see, patients and staff members wheedle, argue, persuade, bargain, negotiate, holler at,

shriek at, command, manipulate relevant contingencies, and attempt to deceive. Additionally, to get jobs done despite the patient's pain, the staff may plainly use force when all other tactics have failed, just as the patient, angry over the staff's failure to relieve the pain, may sign out of the hospital(10).

Clearly, their research shows that in pain management goals and power are not always shared by helper and receiver. In some cases, the staff holds so much power that the patient, in angry frustration, sees that the best alternative is to "sign out" of the relationship.

Further, Fagerhaugh and Strauss point out that the staff expects the patient to cooperate with painful but necessary procedures.

If it is judged necessary that a patient wait for relief, then the patient must endure properly. "Enduring properly" has at least three components. First, the amount and kind of expression of pain should be appropriate to the amount and kind of pain that actually exists. Second, the patient must try to wait until the designated time for relief rather that rushing the staff as it carries on other business. Third, expression of pain should not interfere with any main task being performed in the patient's behalf(10, p. 135).

KOAN

What tactics do nurses use to deal with patients who do not exhibit pain behaviors consistent with their Anglo-American expectations? What other situations can you identify in which there is an imbalance of nurse-patient power? How do you deal with patients whose behaviors do not conform to your cultural expectations of the patient role?

CARE TAKERS AND RISK TAKERS

How does a care taker differ from a risk taker? Both can have and use large amounts of power, influence, and prestige. Both can acquire their positions through legitimate means such as election or through other means such as appointment by an influential friend or relative. Both exhibit power, affiliation, and achievement motivation. The differences between care takers and risk takers are seen in their perspectives and values relative to these motivations (Table 3-1).

KOAN

For an interesting perspective, compare Table 3-1 with the manager-leader characteristics in Table 2-2. Can you add other characteristics of care takers and risk takers to Table 3-1?

What do risk takers and care takers do when they find themselves in the unhappy position of dealing with a crisis of conscience within their organization? Most top government officials choose to leave the organization quietly. Probably most nurses who disagree with their employers also leave silently. The risk takers who make noise are labeled "rebels" and tend to change jobs more often than the acquiesent care takers, although their job changes

---

Table 3–1. Differences Between Care Takers and Risk Takers

Care Taker	Risk Taker
Achievement motives deal with maintaining the status quo	Achievement motives deal with creating and participating in change
Is a team player; conforms to group norms and is loyal to them	Is loyal to own values and principles
Keeps silent when disagreeing with superiors	Voices differences with superiors

are not always voluntary. Dismissed risk takers may find comfort in the adage, "He who appeases the alligator is eaten last."

May sees the care taker and risk taker dichotomy as inevitable: "No matter how much society is changed—and much of it cries to heaven for change—there still will exist the fundamental dialetical situation of individuation against the conformist, leveling tendencies of society"(1, p. 229).

Does the conflict between conformist care takers and nonconformist risk takers occur within the nursing system? Do the risk takers usually accomplish their goals? What criteria determine the outcome, that is, who wins and who loses? Sometimes when it looks as if the rebels have lost, in actuality, they have won or at least have succeeded in bringing an important issue to the public's view. Perhaps more important are the personal rewards.

The rebel insists that his identity be respected; he fights to preserve his intellectual and spiritual integrity against the suppressive demands of society. He must range himself against the group which represents to him conformism, adjustment, and the death of his own originality and voice(1, pp. 225–226).

KOAN

In a small, rural hospital, the chief surgeon had a habit of not taking a history from and giving a physical examination to patients before surgery. The hospital's policy was that the nurse had to sign a paper stating what preoperative preparation was done, including whether the history and physical examination had been done by the surgeon. She tried signing "not done" and was rebuked by the surgeon, who told her that this action was legally dangerous to him and to the hospital. The nurse decided that the best approach was to call the surgeon after each client was admitted for surgery to remind him about the history and physical examination. Each time he told her, "It's been dictated." Most of the time it had not been. The nurse decided that continuation of this behavior was dangerous for providers and clients, so she reported it to her supervisor, who told her that Dr. Z. was an excellent surgeon and that she shouldn't "rock the boat." The nurse then went to the director of nursing, who agreed with her concerns and took the situation to the administrator, who put an immediate halt to Dr. Z.'s behavior.

Think of other situations where a fear of rocking the boat silenced people. Who won? Who lost? Is the win-lose model too simplistic for these types of situations?

In schools of nursing and in nursing literature, nurses are imbued with their responsibility to serve as change agents in the nursing and health care systems. No change can occur without rocking someone's boat, however, and resistance to change is universal (see Chap. 1). Is it ethical and realistic to teach and encourage nurses to change the system without detailing the powerful forces that work against change? Any discussion of risk taking should include the possible dangers of being a rebel in terms of damage to reputation, decreased job opportunities, and an erratic career. The change-agent role often contradicts the traditional image of the nurse as an angel of mercy.

NURSING SYSTEM'S SELF-CONCEPT—ANGELS OF MERCY

After asking me to recommend a head nurse for a hospital and enumerating at length the qualities she must possess to be successful, he concluded with the words, "In short, we require an intelligent saint"(11).

Self-concept and self-esteem have a strong influence on much of a person's behavior. How do nurses view themselves and the services they provide? The Cherry Ames series of novels that first appeared in the 1940s stressed the beautiful Ms. Ames' idealism and commitment. Even though she was having a romantic interaction with an attractive young physician, Cherry Ames "rose respectfully when the physician entered the ward, she always did as she was told, and she was valued by the doctor as 'his' good, concerned nurse"(12). Table 3-2 reflects how some nursing leaders view nurses and nursing.

KOAN

For its graduation ceremony, a class of nurses asked a noted local nurse with no affiliation to appear as the keynote speaker. She agreed without asking for or being offered a fee. The students planned to pay her what was left from their budget, which in the end amounted to nothing, after paying for the organist, supplies, and food for the reception. The class nursing advisor was angry and embarrassed that the students paid the organist but not the nurse/speaker.

Does this incident indicate a low self-esteem among the new nursing graduates? Would the organist have rendered his services for no fee? What would you have done if you were the nurse speaker? What would you have done if you were the class advisor?

A new graduate wrote the following to her former teacher: "I go to work ready to do my best, but I'm not eager. I keep my patients safe, do standard care correctly, pass meds—but I no longer feel able to give of *myself*. And I'm not generating any critical or creative thinking. Not good nursing"(13). Was this nurse socialized during her education to be an "intelligent saint" and an "angel of mercy?" What factors contributed to her dissatisfaction? The problems encountered by this new nurse emphasize the different expectations and self-concepts of the nursing student and of the working nurse. School is one cultural setting while work is another. The differences identified by Kramer and Schmalenberg are listed in Table 3-3(18).

Table 3–2. Nursing Leaders on Nursing's Self-Concept

The old image of nursing was *care of people.* I now see it as becoming the *new* image of nursing.

Lulu K. Wolf Hassenplug (14, p. 113)

I think it is important for today's thinkers about nursing education to know where nursing came from: confined, controlled, narrow, provincial, ordered; illuminated by intense desire to help sick people, self-abnegating; often unaware of its low image.

Lucille Petry Leone (14, p. 168)

I see another crucial issue to be nursing's tendency to react to changes rather than help design them. If we had less internal dissension, we'd have a lot of political clout, and in our society political clout is the name of the game. We're not yet in a position to play that game as national health insurance, quality controls, PSRO's, and other major developments come tumbling out of Washington. If nursing could get itself together and provide the public with a well-defined redefinition of the role of nursing in modern society—what it ought to be—we couldn't fail, given our large numbers. But we wait to see whether the physicians are going to pay or whether hospital administrators will accept our plans.

Mary Kelly Mullane (14, p. 253)

We have large numbers of nurses who would prefer to leave nursing to be physician's assistants. We have an amount of antieducationalism that sometimes seems almost overwhelming. We have large numbers of nurses who deny that there is anything to know in nursing. We have people who are selling nursing right down the river with such weird euphemisms as "pediatric associate" and "primary care practicioner," and so forth.

Martha E. Rogers (14, p. 320)

I continued to be too easily satisfied—not keenly observant— hazy, rather dreary—not sufficiently vigilant—too optimistic—I continued to wish only to do things I liked—my feelings for patients were compassion, or commiseration, or sympathy, rather than a warm personal care. . . . I never began to *think* until I went to Henry Street, and lived with Miss Wald. I was then about 38 years old.

Lavina Dock (15)

Table 3-2. *(Continued)*

I learned from this experience—and many others—that everything one hears about nurses being willing to invest a great deal of effort in patients has to be taken with a grain of salt. . . . In most cases, the resistance to change is not from others; it is from nurses themselves, both from within the systems that I was trying to change and certainly from without.

Luther Christman (16)

Nursing, perhaps more than any other profession, has been influenced by social conceptions regarding the nature of women. Modern nursing originated at a time when Victorian ideas dictated that the role of women was to serve men's needs and convenience. Nursing's development continued to be greatly influenced by the attitudes that women were less independent, less capable of initiative, and less creative than men, and thus need masculine guidance.

JoAnn Ashley (17)

Table 3-3. Comparison of Education and Work Cultures

	Student	Nurse
Rewarded For	Achieving explicit objectives usually related to individual patient care	Achieving implicit objectives many of which are related to organization maintenance and to care of large groups of patients
Organization of Work	Responsible for whole task	Delegation of work and performance of many parts of tasks and few whole tasks
Thinking	Board, cosmopolitan principles	Particulars related to work and their local interpretation

The authors term the conflict between the two systems (each with their own expectations, values, and patterns of communication) as reality shock. They developed the Bicultural Training Program (BTP) to help newly graduated nurses gain interpersonal competence in the nursing subculture of work. Their extensive research found that new graduates who participated in their program had a better understanding of their roles and demonstrated more bicultural role behaviors. Although informal reports from supervisors and peers indicated that the new graduates who had participated in the BTP were adjusting to work better, no statistically significant difference in scores on adjustment tests was found between the group who had BTP and the group that did not. However, more nurses in the BTP program were involved as change agents, resigned less frequently, and received better evaluations(18, p. 3).

KOAN

Do you agree that the cultural setting of nursing education is different from the nursing work setting? Can you identify differences between the two other than those mentioned in Table 3-3? Can you identify other ways of bridging the gap than BTP?

NURSING AND THE FEMINIST MOVEMENT

A look at nursing's self-concept is incomplete without a look at the impact of the feminist movement on nursing. Corea sees nursing as a female occupation controlled from the beginning by males outside the profession. "Doctors controlled nursing effortlessly because it was largely a female occupation. The women had been programmed from childhood to esteem themselves lowly, to assert themselves rarely, to fear power, to shun leadership, to slight their careers. Their minds had been thoroughly conditioned for domination"(4, p.60). Because of the socialization of women, doctor-nurse games were patterned naturally after female-male relationships. Nurses themselves have often been intolerant of other nurses including Margaret Sanger, whose life work had great impact on society but who did not allow themselves to be forced into the traditional female stereotyped behaviors. Women who functioned as lay healers in earlier times did not submit to male domination, but when scientific medicine evolved, nurses were assigned to the caring role while doctors assumed the curing role and received credit for the patient's recovery(19). In light of this, it is interesting to note discussions elsewhere in this book that call for a balance between technology and caring in the holistic health model. Some physicians who recognize the value of caring now see themselves as taking a holistic approach. Will this result in a blurring of physician-nurse roles and thus a blurring of traditional male-female roles?

"Although the worlds of nursing and feminism share similarities in their historical and current problems, neither has attempted to understand, include, or collaborate with the other" (20). Evidence of increasing tolerance for and support of the women's movement is found in the ANA's decision not to hold conventions in states that have not ratified the Equal Rights Amendment. That decision was made by the ANA board of directors after convention delegates defeated a similar resolution.

Angels of Mercy to Queen Bees

The term *Queen Bee syndrome* has evolved in the feminist movement to describe antifeminist behavior in women who have careers in leadership positions. The Queen Bee performs successfully in two roles that appear to be in conflict: the career female role, and the traditional female role. In the work setting, the Queen Bee aligns herself with males and seeks their approval, while in an attempt to reduce competition, she requires women who report to her to perform in the traditional female role, which leads to increased frustration among these women. The Queen Bee may function in either of two ways. She may work very hard to improve the organization supporting change when necessary, but the organization will suffer because she does not train subordinates or share her expertise with them. Or she may work to maintain the status quo, being afraid to risk change. In either case, the Queen Bee has a negative effect on an institution. Realizing that success depends on the values of those in leadership positions, Halsey researched the Queen Bee syndrome in nursing. She found that the Queen Bee syndrome is present in nursing and observed that the "Queen Bee syndrome becomes more prominent in progressively higher levels of nursing management"(21). The Queen Bee syndrome also affects nursing by denying young nurses effective role models and by frustrating aspiring nurse managers in their search for support systems, in the fulfillment of their need for sharing experiences, and in their attempts to institute change.

Even though nursing is beginning to support some of the goals of the feminist movement, nurses have not always been successful when they worked together for a common goal. A recent lawsuit made this painfully clear. Nurses employed by the city of Denver sued for discrimination on the basis of sex(22). The nurses claimed that they were, as a group, paid less than men with similar skills and education and that this type of occupational discrimination has occurred for centuries. The judge was sympathetic and agreed that the nurses' lawsuit had established that male-dominated occupations probably pay more for comparable work than do female-dominated occupations. The judge ruled, however, that there is no law that requires parity of salaries among different occupational groups on the basis of skill required, productivity, or any other criteria, and added that if such a law were enacted, it would precipitate a chaotic restructuring of our economic system(22). The Denver nurses have appealed the decision.

How have women fared in the male-dominated medical profession? In the past, medical schools argued that it was better to admit men than women, since the dropout rate for women was higher and since women were less productive because they practiced fewer hours than men. The number of women in medical schools has risen from about 6% of total enrollment in 1960 to about 28% currently and the dropout rate is equal to, not greater, than that for male students(23). Because the government finances a good deal of medical education and because medical schools found that they could not deny admission to qualified women and remain eligible for federal funds, medical schools changed their policies regarding admission of women. The government's requirements resulted from the feminist movement.

However, women in medicine are in a very difficult position. In addition to dealing with problems posed by marriage and family responsibilities, women in medicine are expected by other women to work to improve medical care while being minority members of a group where the other members have the power.

KOAN

After working in hospital Y for three months as a nursing supervisor, you find that another supervisor with less experience, fewer years of education, and the same responsibilities has a salary of $2,500 more a year than you do. The other supervisor is a man. What would you do?

ACCOUNTABILITY

"Nurses have a unique task before them—the establishment of nursing as an accountable and autonomous profession"(24). Accountability and autonomy are issues receiving much attention in nursing literature. Most nurses who address these issues agree that the nursing system has not achieved autonomy or accepted accountability. Ashley identified several reasons for this: *(1)* nurses have been preoccupied with keeping the economic institution that employs them operating, *(2)* nursing leaders have been too eager to cooperate with existing systems, *(3)* few nursing leaders have been willing to fight publicly for the profession, and *(4)* many nurses have been secure and comfortable in dependent positions where decisions are made for them(17, pp. 125–128).

Health care organizations differ from other organizations in that the majority of their labor force, in theory, is professionally autonomous. In reality, however, physicians control much of the decision-making and activities of other professionals within the organization. Physicians also control access to the services of the organization. This control over the hospital's "purse strings" has led to extraordinarily powerful positions for physicians. As the revised golden rule says, "He who has the gold makes the rules."

What is autonomy? It is the freedom to make decisions and to control important aspects of the work for which the professional has been educated. Absolute freedom is rare or, perhaps, nonexistent. Even the autonomous physicians rely on the support of other health care professionals, from laboratory technicians to nurses, to provide the proper care for their patients. Autonomy is also influenced by the values or ethics of the professional group, by the laws governing the profession, and by the guidelines set up by peers.

Every professional group has a code of ethics that reflects the values of the group and are designed to regulate the professional behavior of members of the group. Ethical codes are not laws, however, and the enforcers of such codes are the members of professional organizations who may be reluctant to censure a member or who may not consider promulgation of the code of ethics a high priority. Patients' bills of rights are basically ethical standards for health care providers. Listed in Table 3-4 are the American Hospital Association's Bill of Rights; Table 3-5 is a model patients' bill of rights published by the American Civil Liberties Union; and Table 3-6 lists the ANA Code of Ethics for nurses.

KOAN

What similarities and differences do you find among the three standards? What areas are covered in each set of guidelines? Which set of guidelines do you use in your practice?

Laws controlling professional practice are another safeguard against the absolute autonomy of the profession. Each state has its own statutes governing the practice of nursing. Nurse practice acts include definitions of nursing, qualifications for licensure, statements concerning reciprocity, powers and composition of the state board of nursing, limitations on the practice of nursing, requirements for license renewal, grounds for license denial, suspension, revocation and probation, injunctive proceedings, and the determination of the necessity for continuing nursing education(26). The state boards of nursing are usually charged with

Table 3–4. American Hospital Association: A Patient's Bill of Rights

The American Hospital Association presents a Patient's Bill of Rights with the expectation that observance of these rights will contribute to more effective patient care and greater satisfaction for the patient, his physician, and the hospital organization. Further, the Association presents these rights in the expectation that they will be supported by the hospital on behalf of its patients, as an integral part of the healing process. It is recognized that a personal relationship between the physician and the patient is essential for the provision of proper medical care. The traditional physician-patient relationship takes on a new dimension when care is rendered within an organizational structure. Legal precedent has established that the institution itself also has a responsibility to the patient. It is in recognition of these factors that these rights are affirmed.

1. The patient has the right to considerate and respectful care.

2. The patient has the right to obtain from his physician complete current information concerning his diagnosis, treatment, and prognosis in terms the patient can be reasonably expected to understand. When it is not medically advisable to give such information to the patient, the information should be made available to an appropriate person in his behalf. He has the right to know, by name, the physician responsible for coordinating his care.

3. The patient has the right to receive from his physician information necessary to give informed consent prior to the start of any procedure and/or treatment. Except in emergencies, such information for informed consent should include but not necessarily be limited to the specific procedure and/or treatment, the medically significant risks involved, and the probable duration of incapacitation. Where medically significant alternatives for care or treatment exist, or when the patient requests information concerning medical alternatives, the patient has the right to such information. The patient also has the right to know the name of the person responsible for the procedures and/or treatment.

4. The patient has the right to refuse treatment to the extent permitted by law and to be informed of the medical consequences of his action.

5. The patient has the right to every consideration of his privacy concerning his own medical care program. Case discussion, consultation, examination, and treatment are confidential and should be conducted discreetly. Those

not directly involved in his care must have the permission of the patient to be present.

6. The patient has the right to expect that all communications and records pertaining to his care should be treated as confidential.

7. The patient has the right to expect that within its capacity a hospital must make reasonable response to the request of a patient for services. The hospital must provide evaluation, service, and/or referral as indicated by the urgency of the case. When medically permissible, a patient may be transferred to another facility only after he has received complete information and explanation concerning the needs for and alternatives to such a transfer. The institution to which the patient is to be transferred must first have accepted the patient for transfer.

8. The patient has the right to obtain information as to any relationship of his hospital to other health care and educational institutions insofar as his care is concerned. The patient has the right to obtain information as to the existence of any professional relationships among individuals, by name, who are treating him.

9. The patient has the right to be advised if the hospital proposes to engage in or perform human experimentation affecting his care or treatment. The patient has the right to refuse to participate in such research projects.

10. The patient has the right to expect reasonable continuity of care. He has the right to know in advance what appointment times and physicians are available and where. The patient has the right to expect that the hospital will provide a mechanism whereby he is informed by his physician or a delegate of the physician of the patient's continuing health care requirements following discharge.

11. The patient has the right to examine and receive an explanation of his bill regardless of source of payment.

12. The patient has the right to know what hospital rules and regulations apply to his conduct as a patient.

No catalog of rights can guarantee for the patient the kind of treatment he has a right to expect. A hospital has many functions to perform, including the prevention and treatment of disease, the education of both health professionals and patients, and the conduct of clinical research. All these activities must be conducted with an overriding concern for the patient, and, above all, the recognition of his dignity as a human being. Success in achieving this recognition assures success in the defense of the rights of the patient.

Table 3–5. A Model Patient's Bill of Rights[a]

Preamble: As you enter this health care facility, it is our duty to remind you that your health care is a cooperative effort between you as a patient and the doctors and the hospital staff. During your stay a patients' rights advocate will be available to you. The duty of the advocate is to assist you in all the decisions you must make and in all situations in which your health and welfare are at stake. The advocate's first responsibility is to help you understand the role of all who will be working with you, and to help you understand what your rights as a patient are. Your advocate can be reached at any time of the day by dialing _____ . The following is a list of your rights as a patient. Your advocate's duty is to see to it that you are afforded these rights. You should call your advocate whenever you have any questions or concerns about any of these rights.

1. The patient has a legal right to informed participation in all decisions involving his/her health care program.
2. We recognize the right of all potential patients to know what research and experimental protocols are being used in our facility and what alternatives are available in the community.
3. The patient has a legal right to privacy regarding the source of payment for treatment and care. This right includes access to the highest degree of care without regard to the source of payment for that treatment and care.
4. We recognize the right of a potential patient to complete and accurate information concerning medical care and procedures.
5. The patient has a legal right to prompt attention, especially in an emergency situation.
6. The patient has a legal right to a clear, concise explanation in layperson's terms of all proposed procedures, including the possibilities of any risk of mortality or serious side effects, problems related to recuperation, and probability of success, and will not be subjected to any procedure without his/her voluntary, competent, and understanding consent. The specifics of such consent shall be set out in a written consent form, signed by the patient.
7. The patient has a legal right to a clear, complete, and accurate evaluation of his/her condition and prognosis without treatment before being asked to consent to any test or procedure.
8. We recognize the right of the patient to know the identity and professional status of all those providing service. All personnel have been instructed to introduce themselves, state their status, and explain their role in the health care of the patient. Part of this right is the right of the patient to know the identity of the physician responsible for his/her care.
9. We recognize the right of any patient who does not speak English to have access to an interpreter.

Table 3–5. *(Continued)*

10. The patient has a right to all the information contained in his/her medical record while in the health care facility, and to examine the record on request.
11. We recognize the right of a patient to discuss his/her condition with a consultant specialist, at the patient's request and expense.
12. The patient has a legal right not to have any test or procedure, designed for educational purposes rather than his/her direct personal benefit, performed on him/her.
13. The patient has a legal right to refuse any particular drug, test, procedure, or treatment.
14. The patient has a legal right to privacy of both person and information with respect to: the hospital staff, other doctors, residents, interns and medical students, researchers, nurses, other hospital personnel, and other patients.
15. We recognize the patient's right of access to people outside the health care facility by means of visitors and the telephone. Patients may stay with their children and relatives with terminally ill patients 24 hours a day.
16. The patient has a legal right to leave the health care facility regardless of his/her physical condition or financial status, although the patient may be requested to sign a release stating that he/she is leaving against the medical judgment of his/her doctor or the hospital.
17. The patient has a right not to be transferred to another facility unless he/she has received a complete explanation of the desirability and need for the transfer, the other facility has accepted the patient for transfer, and the patient has agreed to transfer. If the patient does not agree to transfer, the patient has the right to a consultant's opinion on the desirability of transfer.
18. A patient has a right to be notified of his/her impending discharge at least one day before it is accomplished, to insist on a consultation by an expert on the desirability of discharge, and to have a person of the patient's choice notified in advance.
19. The patient has a right, regardless of the source of payment, to examine and receive an itemized and detailed explanation of the total bill for services rendered in the facility.
20. The patient has a right to competent counseling from the hospital staff to help in obtaining financial assistance from public or private sources to meet the expenses of services received in the institution.
21. The patient has a right to timely prior notice of the termination of his/her eligibility for reimbursement by any third-party payer for the expense of hospital care.

Table 3-5. *(Continued)*

22. At the termination of his/her stay at the health care facility we recognize the right of a patient to a complete copy of the information contained in his/her medical record.
23. We recognize the right of all patients to have 24-hour-a-day access to a patient's rights advocate who may act on behalf of the patient to assert or protect the rights set out in this document.

a Reprinted with permission(25).

Table 3-6. ANA Code of Ethics [a]

1. The nurse provides services with respect for human dignity and the uniqueness of the client unrestricted by considerations of social or economic status, personal attributes, or the nature of health problems.
2. The nurse safeguards the client's right to privacy by judiciously protecting information of a confidential nature.
3. The nurse acts to safeguard the client and the public when health care and safety are affected by the incompetent, unethical, or illegal practice of any person.
4. The nurse assumes responsibility and accountability for individual nursing judgments and actions.
5. The nurse maintains competence in nursing.
6. The nurse exercises informed judgment and uses individual competence and qualifications as criteria in seeking consultation, accepting responsibilities, and delegating nursing activities to others.
7. The nurse participates in activities that contribute to the ongoing development of the profession's body of knowledge.
8. The nurse participates in the profession's efforts to implement and improve standards of nursing.
9. The nurse participates in the profession's efforts to establish and maintain conditions of employment conducive to high-quality nursing care.
10. The nurse participates in the profession's effort to protect the public from misinformation and misrepresentation and to maintain the integrity of nursing.
11. The nurse collaborates with members of the health professions and other citizens in promoting community and national efforts to meet the health needs of the public.

a *Code for Nurses with Interpretive Statements* American Nurses' Association 1976. Reprinted with permission of the American Nurses' Association.

establishing safe standards for nursing practice and for the preparation of practitioners. The major functions of the nursing boards are to protect the public from inadequately prepared or unscrupulous nurses. Thus, the main function of state nursing boards is to serve as a consumer advocate group. However, boards of nursing have been under attack lately for not including more consumers on the board and for their monopoly status in setting standards. Some groups are even questioning the value of mandatory licensure.

Florence Nightingale's goals for nursing care included standards for environmental factors such as sanitation. Since her time nurses have set standards for their practice that varied according to local and state or national expectations, but no standards were published and widely distributed until the early 1970s. Specific, well-defined guidelines for nursing practice were first published by the ANA in 1973, including overall standards as well as standards for specific areas of practice. One impetus for the development of these standards was the federal government's enactment of legislation to provide health insurance for the elderly in the mid 1960s, which required documentation that nursing standards were being met. The assumption was that through peer review standards would be implemented. The ANA standards supplement the nurse practice acts as the legal basis for nursing practice. Nurses can supplement the ANA standards by developing specific standards for their special needs if they work in a specialty area.

To whom, then, is the nurse accountable? The nurse is accountable to several different groups. She is accountable to the patient, to the licensing board that represents society, to the profession of nursing, to the employing agency, and to other health professionals for collaborative functions. The confusion and conflict created by the demands of these various groups are highlighted in Chapter 2 and Figure 3-1.

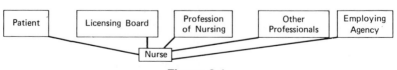

Figure 3-1.

KOAN

Discuss the relationship chart in Figure 3-1 and specify what type of relationship the nurse has with each group. Does the nurse have a relationship of collaboration or legal responsibility with each of the identified groups?

Many nurses still believe they are primarily accountable to the physician under the "Captain-of-the-Ship" doctrine. That doctrine is now recognized as valid in very few situations, such as in the operating room or in the situation when the physician employs the nurse and pays her salary. Current laws stipulate that a nurse who is ordered by a physician to peform an act that in her estimation is unsafe for the patient must refuse to perform the act. The nurse's idea that she is not accountable and can "pass the buck" to the physician is no longer applicable.

Another problem in accountability arises from the fact that experience and educational background vary greatly among nurses. It is unrealistic and unsafe to assume that any nurse can perform any nursing task. Employers have begun to recognize this and so has the ANA, which has developed a credentials program to recognize special skills and knowledge in specified areas of nursing practice.

Since most professional nurses practice within complex systems based on values and goals that may be incongruent with those of the nurses themselves, conflict occurs and a degree of autonomy is lost. This happens in other systems as well. For example, attorneys with liberal political views who work in prominent politically conservative firms are often given the message (however subtle) that their political views should be kept private. The architect designing a public park must satisfy the involved regulations and requirements of government agencies, community groups, and the contractor. In practice, professionals use their expertise to satisfy the varied demands of different consumers of their services.

Once a nurse is committed to working in a system, some of her personal values and goals may come into conflict with the system's values and goals. An example of this in nursing occurred when a senior nursing student on a job interview asked, "What is the difference between the role of staff nurses and the role of practical nurses in this institution?" After some thought, the interviewer, a nurse coordinator, replied, "In our institution practical nurses do not administer medications."

KOAN

Before committing herself to a system, a nurse needs to assess whether the values and goals of the institution conflict with her own. Consider the system you are working in or may work in. How much conflict or incongruence exists between the system's values and your own related to the parameters listed below?

Parameter	System's Values	Nurse's Values
Traditional: refers to the history of roles in the institution		
Hierarchical: refers to organizational structure		
Bureaucratic: refers to rules, policies		
Social: refers to whether or not stratification occurs between and within disciplines		

Parameter	System's Values	Nurse's Values
Political: refers to who holds the power, makes decisions, has input		

System assessment can often be helpful in clarifying for the nurse the degree of congruency that exists between the system's and the nurse's values. Conflict in the professional role is often a result of the mismatch between nurse and system. As nursing continues to develop its research-based body of knowledge, conflict between more slowly evolving systems, such as hospitals, and professional nurses may increase for a time.

RESEARCH DEVELOPMENT: A POWER ISSUE

Prominent nurses and observers of nursing have identified a need for increasing inquiry into the science of nursing and into the development of nursing theory.

> The extent to which nursing can exert social influence through its particular body of knowledge and skills is a function of *(a)* the competence of its practitioners, scholars and new recruits; *(b)* the capacity it may have to bring about positive results in the health status of its clientele; and *(c)* the continued appraisal and extension of that capacity through basic and clinical research, as well as through the activities of related health fields(27).

In 1974, the ANA House of Delegates resolved to "make a concerted effort to build a public image of nursing research as an essential contribution to knowledge in the health care field" with the thrust of the research in the next decade being focused on theories and practice of nursing(28). Emphasis on research in nursing is a new development. Until recently, most nurses based a great deal of their practice on intuition. They knew, usually through experience, what would work and what would not work for particular nursing problems. Similarly, definitions and theories of what nursing is and how its services are provided were based largely on ideas that were not tested scientifically.

Intuitive nursing practice is not acceptable in our technological, scientifically oriented society. "The final quarter of the twentieth century may well see nursing as a major contributor to research in health care. The time is ripe and the work is long overdue"(27, p. 21). Fleming identifies eight developments that indicate that nurses are beginning to accept research as an activity(29):

1. Increase in the number of research articles
2. Establishment of the journal, *Nursing Research*, in 1952
3. Publication of the journal, *Research in Nursing and Health*
4. Designation of the Commission on Nursing Research within the ANA
5. Establishment of the Council on Nurse Researchers within the ANA
6. Increase in the number of positions for nurse researchers in practical and educational settings
7. Inclusion of research content in baccalaureate and masters programs in nursing
8. Establishment of doctoral programs designed to prepare nurse researchers, and increase in the number of nurses entering doctoral programs.

Throughout most of modern nursing's history, nursing practice has been firmly rooted in medical practice. Physicians taught nursing students, and textbooks were organized around medical pathophysiology with physicians as coauthors and/or as major reference sources. In the 1960s, nurses began to recognize the separate and unique aspects of their practice as well as the inadequacies of the medical model as a basis for nursing practice. This was the beginning of the evolution of nursing theory, which is still in its infancy. Three main approaches to the development of nursing theory have emerged during these initial stages: "*(1)* the 'borrowing' of theory from other disciplines with intent to integrate it into a science of nursing; *(2)* an analysis of nursing practice situations in search of the theoretical underpinnings; and *(3)* the creation of a conceptual system from which theories could be derived"(30).

Although all sciences use an established core of knowledge, nurses who try to borrow theories from other disciplines may have difficulty in applying that information to nursing and in using it to generate theory that will expand nursing science.

> Since the primary goal of nursing theory is the generation of knowledge specific to nursing, the process of theory building must be couched in a nursing frame of reference. Otherwise, the obtained knowledge will not be nursing knowledge which can be used to build or expand nursing science or be used for nursing education, practice or research(31).

In its research endeavors, nursing must avoid the research narrowness that some other sciences have experienced. A systems approach can help prevent the situation from arising in which nurse researchers can explain their work only to other nurse researchers interested in the same problems. Nurse researchers must maintain an ability to work and to communicate with all nurses and with researchers in other disciplines.

COLLABORATION: MYTH OR REALITY

Intraprofessional collaboration (among nurses) is taught in basic nursing programs primarily through the team or primary nursing models. The patient care conference is a core component of the team model and is essential for that model to work well. In practice, team conferences are not held frequently. Interprofessional collaboration (among different professions) is also included in the course content of basic nursing programs, and the topic frequently comes up in nursing journals. Is interprofessional collaboration also taught in the basic medical program? In 1973 a state medical association's position on interprofessional relationships stated:

The delivery of optimum health care should be a cooperative effort under the physician's leadership, wherein nurses
and other health care personnel work under his supervision.
An independent, autonomous nurse practitioner is inconsis-
tent with this position and must lead to second-class medical care(32).

Collaboration is different from cooperation. Cooperation means
that one party gives in to the values or goals of another party if
conflict occurs. Collaboration is a reciprocal relationship in which
communication is open and free between two parties. For example, communication patterns look like this A $\rightleftarrows$ B. Ideas, messages, and energy flow freely between the two components involved in communication. Before this can happen, however, both
parties need to understand the purpose and goals of the other and
to respect the other's efforts.

In Table 3-7 are listed some potential positive and negative
effects of collaboration. Can you think of additional potential
positive and negative effects?

Table 3–7. Potential Effects of Collaboration

Positive Effects	Negative Effects
Decreases duplication of efforts	Takes more time than noncollaboration
Challenges each party to examine own practice and values	Decreases competition that may decrease organizational energy and motivation
Increases energy available for task at hand	Either or both parties may resist if (1) don't know or understand goals and values of other party; (2) don't respect the work of the other party; (3) don't respect the work of members of own group
Allows maximum exploitation of resources	
Enhances role performance of each party	One party may have to share its legitimate authority

---

KOAN

In a critical care unit, nurses were experiencing difficulty getting physicians to respond when a patient's condition changed. One nurse, concerned about the patients' welfare and her own liability, complained through appropriate channels of communication in the nursing hierarchy to no avail on several occasions. As her anxiety increased, her complaints became more strident. One day as the attending physician was examining a patient, the nurse blurted her concerns to him. Quickly her supervisor, who was nearby, apologized for the nurse's behavior labeling her as "young and idealistic." The physician disagreed. "Her concerns are valid. She is very realistic. She is the best nurse that you have," he said.

Why did this situation occur? How could it have been prevented? Can you identify some specific methods of dealing with similar problems? For example, would a joint practice committee of the critical care unit nurses and physicians be helpful?

Other examples of decreased collaboration abound. Florence Nightingale collaborated when it suited her goals. But for the most part, she worked independently, communicating her wishes and instructions through letters and directives. Staff nurses may feel uncomfortable about consulting a nursing clinical specialist and using her special knowledge and skills. Nurses in education and those in practice disagree on the purposes and goals of the basic program and on how students are taught. The ANA and the NLN duplicate some efforts and disagree on which organization should do what. Some of these examples of decreased collaboration among nurses are recognized by the parties involved and attempts, not always successful, have been made to increase collaboration. Large-scale attempts to increase collaboration, such as those between the ANA and the NLN, have not been noticeably fruitful. For example, in 1974 the ANA House of Delegates directed ANA to "examine" the feasibility of accreditation of basic and undergraduate education," a function of the NLN(33). Although the ANA invited the NLN to participate in its study, the NLN declined, citing serious questions about the study design (34).

Collaboration in Hierarchical Systems

Hospitals are formally organized according to the bureaucratic model, which has four characteristics: a clear-cut division of labor, a system of controls, a method of assigning roles based on technical qualifications, and a carefully structured hierarchy. In recent years, the term *bureaucracy* has developed a negative connotation. There are, however, advantages to bureaucracies. Although employees are often too closely supervised within bureaucracies, bureaucratic systems "ensure that officials are limited in the facets of their subordinates they control and how they may exercise that control"(35).

The informal organizational structure of the bureaucracy complements the formal hierarchy through its flexibility and spontaneity and its ability to provide a sense of belonging and security to employees in the work setting. The manager's role is made simpler if it is supported by the informal organization, and the informal organization can provide an additional source of communication, the grapevine, for the bureaucracy(35, p. 66). Occasionally, the informal organization and the bureaucracy work at cross purposes, which creates problems for the worker.

The formal and informal organizations of a hospital must be balanced, and nurses should be equally aware of the workings of both. Nursing, however, with its roots in religious and military systems, often operates "by the book" and fails to integrate a knowledge of the informal organization into its development of strategy. Understanding all aspects of the system, planning strategy, and exploiting resources are critical elements in successful problem-solving. Nurses may not have the necessary skills to function this way.

Traditional worship of authority, still sometimes inculcated through the educational process, the socialization of the young nurse in the mores of the institution, the reliance on those above to make the right decision, the fear of questioning and generating open controversy—all combine historically and currently for political naivete in nurses as a class(36).

KOAN

Nurses in a certain hospital were required to wear their caps at all times. The nurses in the critical care unit protested to their supervisors in the bureaucratic hierarchy that caps were awkward and interfered with patient care. The director of nursing was firm: All nurses will wear caps. One day during cardiopulmonary resuscitation of a patient, a physician was poked in the eye with a nurses cap. He angrily directed the nurse to remove her cap, and he went to the director of nursing as soon as the emergency had ended. After telling his story, he demanded that caps be forbidden in the critical care unit. The director of nursing agreed and caps were banished from the critical care unit.

Was this a success for the bureaucracy or for the informal organization? Why? Can you identify resources that the nurses could have mobilized in their first attempts to institute change?

Nursing is ambivalent regarding collaboration and rightly so. On the one hand, nursing cries for unity among diverse educational groups, and, on the other hand, continually cites a crisis in leadership involving those very leaders who have been able to decrease the divisiveness among these groups. It may be wise to remember that the greatest leaders in science and history have gone it alone. Freud, Darwin, Einstein, Salk, and Nightingale did not convene committees to accomplish their goals. While collaboration is necessary in that it helps a system function smoothly, conflict is useful in developing leadership and encouraging creativity.

CONFLICT RESOLUTION

Although collaboration generally creates few, if any, emotional reactions, conflict inevitably does. Conflict occurs between two independent parties on issues important to both that reflect their value systems. Conflict can be constructive or destructive. Kramer and Schmalenberg identify four types of conflict(18, pp. 255–256):

1. *Professional-bureaucratic:* due to incompatible expectations from the bureaucracy and the profession
2. *Means-goals:* due to lack of a known means to achieve desired goals
3. *Personal competency:* due to lack of skill or knowledge
4. *Expressive-instrumental:* due to differences in the individual's conceptions of appropriate role behavior

All participants in the nursing system have experienced conflict at some time. Using Kramer and Schmalenberg's framework for classifying types of conflict, it is easy to think of an example of a conflict in each category. Cost-cutting measures that lead to decreased staffing occur in the professional-bureaucratic category. Means-goals conflicts are reflected in the nursing system's inability to develop adequate tools to evaluate the quality of nursing care. Nurses asked to perform tasks for which they are not prepared experience a personal competency conflict. How many nurses have been asked to cover ICU "because we're understaffed and you're better than no nurse at all?" Role-expectation conflicts can occur between any parts of the system from patient-nurse conflicts to conflicts between nurses and other professionals. A patient who demands immediate response to his or her needs and criticizes the busy nurse's priorities exemplifies the role-expectation conflict. These are only a few of the many conflicts a nurse is confronted with; she may be confronted with all four at one time! How do these and other conflicts get resolved? Conflict resolution can be a source of growth and provide personal satisfaction or it can be frustrating and disruptive. Conflict as a source of growth or as a disruptive influence is illustrated in Figure 3-2, which was developed from many sources, the major one being Low (37).

To resolve conflict successfully with a physician over a medication error, for instance, the nurse can petition the system to hold joint meetings between physicians and nurses for problem-solving and facilitating communication. The nurse can then suggest that physicians and nurses openly challenge each other's

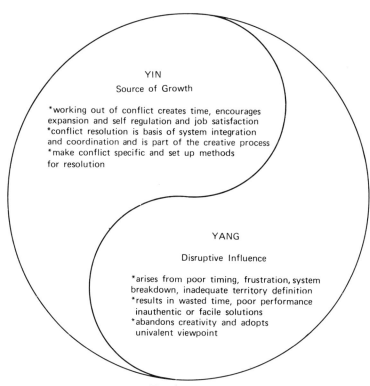

Figure 3-2.

clinical judgments and resolve differences on clinical grounds. To aid her own functioning in conflict situations with physicians, the nurse can learn assertive communication techniques, find a role model who manages conflict and collaboration well and study her in action, and encourage patients to be their own advocates in dealings with the physician(38).

From their study of conflicts in nursing, Kramer and Schmalenberg made some suggestions: "nursing needs to develop a positive, constructive attitude toward conflict" and an "awareness of our skills in conflict resolution"(19, p.3). Further research is needed about the types of conflict encountered by nurses so that patient care and nurse job satisfaction can improve.

KOAN

Remember a recent conflict situation in which you were involved. Recreate the arguments you used in the situation and analyze those arguments using the yin (source of growth) and yang (disruptive influence) model.

Conflict and Decision-Making

What effect does conflict have on the decision-making process? In studying decision-making behavior in nurse leaders, for example, Taylor found that the leaders were more concerned with the quality of a decision than with its acceptance by their subordinates. Furthermore, the leaders tended not to use the group process when conflict was built into decision-making situations. Rather, they used more autocratic decision-making processes(39). In other words, in high conflict situations, nurse leaders did not resort to collaboration.

Janis and Mann have identified five stages in the decision-making process(40).

Stage	Key Questions
1. Appraising the challenge	Are the risks serious if I don't change?

Stage	*Key Questions*
2. Surveying the alternatives	Is this salient alternative an acceptable means for dealing with the challenge? Have I sufficiently surveyed the available alternatives?
3. Weighing the alternatives	Which alternative is best? Could the best alternative meet the essential requirements?
4. Deliberations about commitment	Shall I implement the best alternative and allow others to know?
5. Adhering despite negative feedback	Are the risks serious if I don't change? Are the risks serious if I do change?

The nurse leader's leanings toward the authoritarian style raises the question: What impact does managerial style have on conflict resolution and decision-making? Maccoby has identified four types of leaders and their values in decision-making or conflict resolution(41).

Type of Leader	*Values in Decision-Making and Conflict Resolution*
Craftsperson	Traditional values. Enjoys building. Perfectionist. Self-contained. Tends to do own thing. Few are successful managers. Needs protected nest at work and home.
Jungle fighter	Goal is power. Views peers as accomplices or enemies and subordinates as objects to be used. Can be "lion" who conquers or "fox" who advances by politicking.
Company person	Identity based on being part of powerful, protective company. Concerned with human side of company, feelings of people, and organization's integrity. Creative ones create cooperation, stimulation, mutuality. Less creative ones find a niche.

Type of Leader	Values in Decision-Making and Conflict Resolution
Gamesperson	New type of manager. Main interest is challenge, competitive activity, winning. Likes risks. Views life and work as a game. Energizes others through enthusiasm.

Combinations of these four types of leaders occur, and all four types are needed to make an organization work with the exception of the jungle fighter, which most organizations can function without. In what category or combination of categories do the nurse managers you are familiar with belong?

Leaders use one of five methods for making decisions(42):

Autocratic I (AI)	You solve the problem or make the decision yourself, using information available to you at the time.
Autocratic II (AII)	You obtain the necessary information from your subordinates, then decide the solution to the problem yourself. You may or may not tell your subordinates what the problem is in getting the information from them. The role played by your subordinates in making the decision is clearly one of providing the necessary information to you, rather than of generating or evaluating alternative solutions.
Consultative I (CI)	You share the problem with the relevant subordinates individually, getting their ideas and suggestions without bringing them together as a group. Then you make the decision, which may or may not reflect your subordinates' influence.
Consultative II (CII)	You share the problem with your subordinates as a group, obtaining their collective ideas and suggestions. Then you make the decision, which may or may not reflect your subordinates' influence.

Group II (GII)   You share the problem with your subordinates as a group. Together you generate and evaluate alternatives and attempt to reach agreement (consensus) on a solution. Your role is much like that of chairperson. You do not try to influence the group to adopt your solution, and you are willing to accept and implement any solution that has the support of the entire group.

KOAN

Can you see a correlation between type of leader and method used for decision-making? Match the type of leader with the decision-making method that seems most appropriate for that leader.

In your experience, nurse leaders use which type of decision-making method? Which method are you most comfortable with?

Managing Conflict

Managing conflict must begin with an assessment of self and of the conflict situation and an examination of feelings about conflict and expectations related to the conflict. Assessment progresses to examination of rewards within the system for collaboration and conflict resolution. If the system does not reward conflict resolution, are there other rewards for solving the conflict? Is communication open, honest, assertive, contemplated? Or is it defensive, threatening, emotional? What is the issue? In some situations, such as means-goals conflicts, where no known answers are available, the conflict may have to be resolved through agreement that there is no answer. Finally, the assessment examines leadership styles, power alliances, and decision-making styles of involved parties. Consider this case of conflict:

Dr. Smith came to the Intensive Care Unit to make surgical rounds. He was accompanied by two surgical residents. As he approached Mr. Diehl's bed, he saw Ms. Jones changing a soiled CVP dressing according to the procedure-book guidelines. The following conversation occurred:

Dr. Smith (sarcastically): "I don't know what to do with her! (the nurse). I should either throw her out of the unit or bang her against the wall! I don't want anyone touching my dressings!"

Ms. Jones: "Is something wrong?"

Dr. Smith: "You dumb nurses never follow instructions. I've said it a hundred times. Don't touch my dressings."

By this time the conversation was so loud that it was disrupting the other patients, so the head nurse, Mr. George, went to Mr. Diehl's bedside and said to Dr. Smith, "What's wrong here?" To which Dr. Smith yelled, "She changed my dressing. You know that nurses never touch my dressings. I'm going to report this to the nursing office."

Mr. George, the head nurse, answered, "I should be reporting you for screaming at nurses, disrupting the unit, and upsetting patients. If you want to yell, come in the back room, and we'll yell this out." Mr. George then walked away and went to the back room. Dr. Smith left the unit in anger.

This situation represents a bureaucratic-professional and a role-expectation conflict. For some reason, Dr. Smith's directives concerning "his dressings" were not communicated or the nurse changed the soiled dressings because in her judgment they were harmful to the patient's health. Communication was emotional, defensive, and threatening. The head nurse was a combination of the company person, concerned with the feelings of people and the integrity of the organization—and the craftsperson—the perfectionist. His decision-making method was autocratic. He decided to make decisions and solve the problem himself without using other members of his work group. In his decision-making process, did the head nurse examine and weigh alternative ways of handling the conflict? Or did he automatically react to an attack?

If this case were being rewritten as an example of conflict as a source of growth, what changes would be indicated in the characters and the script? Would the head nurse's leadership style and decision-making method be altered? How would the communication pattern change? This nurse and physician might have experienced the conflict as a source of growth if they had used assertive rather than aggressive communication techniques. Another tool that might have been useful in this situation is role clarification and role negotiation.

Leaving conflicts unsuccessfully resolved leads to a reduction in growth, creativity, and ability to do work. Serious conflicts do not "go away" if they are ignored. Suppressed or unresolved conflicts lead to interpersonal hostility and task disruptions that keep the system unbalanced(37). According to Low, "The fear of conflict itself is one of the major causes of poor organization." Through refusing to face and reconcile conflict in a creative way, many managers subsume roles and tasks under departmental heads that should not functionally exist there(37, p. 63).

KOAN

Is the elaborate hierarchy in nursing organizations an attempt to control and minimize conflict?

Rather than retreat from conflict, nurses can use conflict as a challenge to develop new skills in communicating and collaborating. Conflict can be a stimulus for nurses to examine their perspectives and develop new perspectives. This challenge to creativity, if met, can be deeply satisfying to the nurse both as a person and as a professional.

REFERENCES

1. May R: *Power and Innocence: A Search for the Sources of Violence.* New York, W W Norton & Co Inc., 1972, p 99.

2. McClelland DC: *Power: The Inner Experience.* New York, Irvington Publishers Inc, 1975, p 14.

3. Seigler M, Osmond H: Aesculapian authority. *Hastings Center Studies* 1:44, 1973.

4. Corea G: *The Hidden Malpractice: How American Medicine Treats Women As Patients and Professionals.* New York, William Morrow & Co Inc, 1977.

5. *Am J Nurs* 78:1824, 1978.

6. Getting involved in politics: A how-to-do-it guide. Nurses Coalition for Action in Politics 1978, p 5.

7. Collins E, Scott P: Everyone who makes it has a mentor: Interviews with F.J. Lunding, G.L. Clements and D.S. Perkins. *Harvard Business Review* 56:90, 1978.

8. Schorr TM: The lost art of mentorship, editorial. *Am J Nurs* 78:1873, 1978.

9. Leininger M: *Transcultural Nursing: Concepts, Theories and Practices.* New York, John Wiley & Sons Inc, 1978, p 11.

10. Fagerhaugh S, Strauss A: *Politics of Pain Management: Staff Patient Interaction.* Menlo Park, California, Addison-Wesley Publishing Co Inc, 1977, p 8.

11. Robb IH: *Nursing Ethics: For Hospital and Private Use.* Cleveland, E.C. Koeckert, 1900, p40.

12. Hott JH: Updating Cherry Ames. Am J Nurs 77:1581, 1977.

13. Miller S: Letter from a new graduate. *Am J Nurs* 78:1688, 1978.

14. Safier G: *Contemporary American Leaders in Nursing: An Oral History,* New York, McGraw-Hill, 1977.

15. Dock L: Self Portrait, *Nursing Outlook* 25:25, 1977.

16. Lysaught J: "Christmas Present: An Interview on a Life's Career in Nursing Leadership." *Nursing Digest,* VI:2, 6, 1978.

17. Ashley J: *Hospitals, Paternalism and the Role of the Nurse.* New York, Teachers College Press, 1977, pp 75–76.

18. Kramer M, Schmalenberg C: *Path to Biculturalism.* Wakefield, Massachusetts, Contemporary Publishing Inc, 1977, pp 113, 129–137.

19. Ehrenreich B, English D: *Witches, Midwives and Nurses: A History of Women Healers.* Old Westbury, New York, 40–41 Feminist Press, 1973.

20. Kritek P, Glass L: Nursing: A feminist perspective. *Nurs Outlook.* 26:182, 1978.

21. Halsey S: The queen bee syndrome: One solution to role conflict for nurse managers, Hardy M, Conway M (eds): *Role Theory: Perspectives for Health Professionals.* New York, Appleton-Century-Crofts, 1978, p 246.

22. *Lemons et al vs the City and County of Denver.* U.S. District Court, District of Colorado, 1978 No 76-W-1156.

23. Walsh M: *Doctors Wanted: No Women Need Apply.* New Haven, Yale University Press, 1977, 156.

24. Christman L: Accountability and autonomy are more than rhetoric. *Nurse Educ* 3:4, 1978.

25. Annas GJ: The hospital: A human rights wasteland. *The Civil Liberties Review.* 1:21–22.

26. Ceisla J: Nursing practice acts. *Occup Health Nurs,* October 1977, p 13.

27. Gortner S: Trends and historical perspective in Downs F, Fleming J (eds): *Issues in Nursing Research.* New York, Appleton-Century-Crofts, 1979, p 1.

28. "Resolution on Priorities in Nursing Research." *American Nurse,* August 1974, p 6.

29. Fleming J: The future of nursing research, Downs F, Fleming J, (eds): in *Issues in Nursing Research.* New York, Appleton-Century-Crofts, 1979, pp 150–151.

30. Newman M: Nursing's theoretical evolution. *Nurs Outlook* 20:450, 1972.

31. Phillips JR: Nursing systems and nursing models. *Image* 9:4, 1977.

32. *Bull NY Acad Med* 53:501–502, 1977.

33. ANA House of Delegates Convention '74 *AJN* 74:1259.

34. *NLN News* 24:2, 1976.

35. Kohn M: Benefits of bureaucracy. *Human Nature* 1:66, 1978.

36. Kalisch B, Kalisch P: A discourse on the politics of nursing, *J Nurs Adm* 6:30, 1976.

37. Low, A: *Zen and Creative Management.* Garden City, New York, Anchor Books, 1976, p. 60–68.

38. Stanley L: Nurses vs. doctors: What to do when the MD is wrong. *RN* 42:30, 1979.

39. Taylor A: Decision making in nursing: An analytical approach. *J Nurs Adm* November 1978, pp 22–30.

40. Janis I, Mann L: *Decision Making: A Psychological Analysis of Conflict, Choice and Commitment.* New York, The Free Press, 1977, p 172.

41. Maccoby M: *The Gamesman: The New Corporate Leaders.* New York, Simon & Schuster Inc, 1976, p. 46–49.

42. Vroom V, Yetton P: *Leadership and Decision Making.* Pittsburgh, University of Pittsburgh Press, 1973, p 17.

CHAPTER FOUR

The Changing Nursing System

> When a population undergoing drastic change is without abundant opportunities for individual action and self-advancement, it develops a hunger for faith, pride and unity. It becomes receptive to all manner of proselytizing, and is eager to throw itself into collective undertakings which aim at "showing the world." . . . Where things have not changed at all, there is the least likelihood of revolution.
>
> *Eric Hoffer**

CHANGE IN NURSING: REALITY OR ILLUSION

The nursing system is currently preoccupied with change, its meaning, its mechanisms, and its management.

The nursing system is in dynamic interaction with the larger health care delivery system and its rapidly accelerating technology, shifting role-relationships, and underdeveloped ethical models. That the nursing profession is racing headlong into an unknown future may be more illusion than fact. For example, consider the following questions:

*From reference 18.

· How new is the concept of nursing as health maintenance?
· How often have nurses noted that better sanitary conditions, architectural design, and administrative arrangements would facilitate and improve practice?
· How recent is the idea that "light used judiciously has healing properties?"
· How recent are investigations into noise pollution and its effect on the human organism?
· How recent is the concept of man as a psychophysiological unity?
· How old is the idea of sensory deprivation and the person's need for a varied environment?
· How recent is the activity of nursing assessment?

Are these questions five years old? Ten years old? No! Over one hundred years old! Each was treated in considerable depth in Florence Nightingale's *Notes on Nursing* in 1859(1).

However, a glance back through the time spiral at nursing's evolution reveals that the major unresolved issues of yesterday are still problems of the profession. For example, in the late 1800s and early 1900s nursing leaders decried hospital conditions including unsavory sanitary practices, unskilled nursing personnel, poor management, and poor working conditions. Today the nursing system protests dehumanization of care, unrealistic staffing patterns, fiscal mismanagement, and a host of puzzling ethical problems that evolve as rapidly as technology. Same setting, similar issues; different language, different time-frame. The lingering issues of institutional licensure and collective bargaining are expressive of the fundamental question: "Who controls nursing practice?" It might seem that everything has changed, yet nothing has changed.

As a college of nursing faculty meeting was nearing its end, a member reminded the others to contact their congressional representatives concerning the development of a health care credentialing bill that had not had nursing representation or input on the planning committee. Discussion developed concerning federal budget allocations, global goals, and implications for nursing. This particular bill, if

developed, would have grave implications for nurse licensure. Some faculty members loudly expressed dismay that nurses were not represented on such a powerful committee. "Don't be discouraged," said a young faculty member, "nursing is still an emerging profession. Acceptance of our importance to the health care delivery system will come in time." A faculty member who had been a nurse for thirty years laughed, "We were emerging when I was a student thirty-two years ago. When will we finally emerge? When will the egg hatch?"

This discussion between faculty members illustrates the fact that change is a function of perspective. The faculty member who is just starting her career is satisfied with the degree and rate of change that propels nursing toward "emergence" as a distinct discipline or profession. The older faculty member has been through many changes that have only resulted in "more of the same" or "persistence of the system." What is more puzzling is that both are rather accurate in their assessment of the situation.

Change is a powerful but elusive process. Toffler asserts that all "things" are in reality "not things at all but processes"(2). Nowhere in life is there a static point against which to measure change. Change is a constant that may seem paradoxical. It is relative, uneven, and occurs at different rates in different systems.

Toynbee boldly states, "Technology is the only field of human activity in which there has been progression. The advance from Lower Paleolithic to mechanized technology has been immense. There has been no corresponding advance in human sociality, though advances in this field have been called for by the changes in social conditions that have been imposed upon mankind by its technological progress"(3). Toynbee's point is clearly illustrated in nursing practice, where technological change has evolved much more rapidly than social change (Fig. 4-1).

It is not uncommon to find nursing departments readily adjusting to the complexities of staffing a computerized intensive care unit while simultaneously agonizing over whether or not to change traditional hospital dress codes.

The disparity between advanced technological change in nursing practice and traditional role relationships often challenges the decision-making ability and effectiveness of the nurse.

(Figure A)

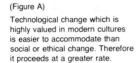

Technological change which is
highly valued in modern cultures
is easier to accommodate than
social or ethical change. Therefore
it proceeds at a greater rate.

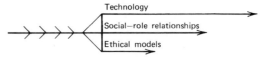

Figure 4-1.

At 11 PM, Nurse M., an experienced and clinically competent nurse, noticed that Mr. G, a 54-year-old man with a pacemaker, had developed a dangerous arrythimia. She notified the medical resident, who was involved in an emergency. He said, "Manage as best you can. I'll be there in ten minutes." Mr. S., a fourth-year medical student, dropped into the unit to read a few charts just as Nurse M. was managing the emergency with Mr. G. The medical student approached the bed. The standard medication administered by the nurse was not effective. Nurse M. readied the defibrillator paddles and just as she was about to act, the medical student shouted authoritatively, "Nurse, don't apply those paddles! You'll blow this man up. He has a pacemaker!" Nurse M. stopped abruptly, looked at the medical student in a perplexed way for several seconds, then reapplied the paddles and defibrillated Mr. G. The patient did not respond nor did he "blow up."

When giving her report at the change of shift, Nurse M. said, "When the medical student shouted at me to stop, I did just that. I had a few seconds of self-doubt. I didn't trust my own experience and judgment. I was thinking, 'He's the doctor and I'm the nurse. He's supposed to know more than I do.' I wonder if those seconds would have made a difference?"

Even though the nursing system has always retained its caring focus, at least on some level, it has moved from an era of hands-on care, applying leeches and administering cathartics to the computerized monitoring and often overreliance on pharmacologic intervention. Like the nurse in the above case, the nursing system continues to struggle in its attempts to strike a balance between caring, nursing's essence, and the impersonal nature of scientific technology.

CHANGE AND TECHNOLOGY

The primacy of technology in bringing the health care delivery system to its present state cannot be overemphasized. The advent of the microscope, the stethoscope, and the thermometer enabled physicians to measure and enumerate the physiologic characteristics of health and disease. As the availability of diagnostic tests and procedures grew in the 1900s, many people in the health care professions worried that the patient was being viewed less as a person and more as an object of study and the doctor more as a research scientist than as a physician.

Reiser tells us that in the United States by the 1930s the new breed of clinical medical professors appeared to be interested primarily in the biochemistry of disease(4). More and more of these research-oriented physicians moved directly from the laboratory into professional clinical chairs in hospitals. The physical examination, which had declined in importance in the medical school curriculum, was often assigned to the younger, less experienced members of the hospital staff. "A number of doctors expressed impatience with the physical examination as imprecise and time-consuming. The laboratory's dramatic discoveries increasingly appeared to diminish the doctor's inclination to use his senses"(4, p. 167).

Reiser points out that among modern physicians a hierarchy of values has emerged that assign greater value to medical evidence obtained through scientific procedures than to data the physician collects with his own senses(4, p. 167). Information volunteered by the patient about his condition is valued even less.

> The physician in the last two centuries has gradually relinquished his unsatisfactory attachment to subjective evidence—what the patient says—only to substitute a devotion to technological evidence—what the machine says. He has thus exchanged one partial view of disease for another. As the physician makes greater use of the technology of diagnosis, he perceives his patient more and more indirectly through a screen of machines and specialists; he also relinquishes his control over more and more of the diagnostic process. These circumstances tend to estrange him from his patient and from his own judgment(4, p. 230).

Conversely, nursing has, through the last 100 years, maintained a more humanistic focus and has become increasingly person- and family-centered in its educational programs and practices. Medicine's disenchantment with history-taking and the physical examination has opened the way for nurses to combine these two important diagnostic tools with a humanistic philosophy to improve the quality of health care. Unlike medicine, nursing is still relatively free from the bondage of technology; although nursing, in some areas, is becoming increasingly technologically oriented.

Technology can seduce the nursing system just as it has the medical system. Technology cannot be denied or ignored. It promises to proliferate, even though it often seems to detract from rather than enhance the caring process. It is important for nurses to integrate technology into caring instead of wishing it would go away so nurses could get "back to basics." When describing practice, the nurse who identifies primarily technologically related tasks has an imbalance and may be one of those seduced by technology.

KOAN

Rank the order (from most important to least important) of these functions performed by nurses:

_____ **Collaborates with other members of health team.**

_____ **Administers medications and parenteral fluids**

_____ **Performs range-of-motion exercises with patient**

_____ **Conducts health teaching**

_____ **Provides emotional support**

_____ **Monitors machines being used on patient (dialysis, cardiac monitors, CVP lines, respirator)**

How does your ordering of these functions relate/correspond to the amount of time each day a nurse spends performing these functions. For

---

example, does the function that is most important take the most time? If an incongruency exists, why is it so? What can be done about this incongruence?

CHANGING TO PERSIST

There is a mystique about change and its paradoxical interdependence with persistence. Buckley reminds us that the continuity, or persistence, of a complex adaptive system such as the nursing system depends on change in its structure. Just as the person must change physiologically and psychologically from minute to minute to survive, so must the nursing system change to endure (5). The degree of change in any system is a "complex function of the *internal state* of the system, the state of its relevant environment and the nature of the interchange between the two" (5, p. 493).

Toynbee points out that societal systems or civilizations evolved not simply because of innate factors or ideal environmental conditions but through a process of challenge (from the environment) and response (according to the state of the system). For example, the sudden crushing defeat of a people is apt "to stimulate the defeated party to set its house in order"(6) and prepare to make a victorious response. The promise of breaking in "new grounds or territory" also has been an impetus for systems to change. Conversely, primitive social systems that remain static for too long do not persist(6).

The same analogies could be applied to the adaptive, open nursing system. Challenge from the environment in the form of plagues and wars were responsible for the formation of some of the great nursing orders of medieval times. Lavinia Dock admitted to having been a rather complacent nurse until she went to work as a visiting nurse at the Henry Street Settlement. There she was "radicalized" as she learned of the lifelong struggles and persecution of the working class(7). The appalling conditions of the military hospitals in the Crimea, and hospital care in general, challenged Nightingale to set a course toward reformation and modernization of nursing and hospital care. Challenge from the environment and the response of a creative minority or person is a recurrent theme in the progress of all human systems throughout history.

KOAN

What challenges are presented to you by the health care delivery systems in which you have been a practitioner, student, observer or client that might set you on a course of changing a part or all of the nursing system or the health care system?

Why should the nursing system change? Why does the nursing rhetoric beckon change? Could it be that the nurse in many instances acts as an agent of persistence instead of an agent of change?

Perhaps nursing is unconsciously yearning for stability and permanence in a chaotic educational and practice system that "through the accident of evolution and our own repeated acts of disunity, we now have"(8). Perhaps, like Hamlet, we would "rather bear those ills we have than fly to others that we know not of."

Change, however, is a pervasive phenomenon, so much so that its nature should be more clearly understood. What is needed is a model for understanding change within systems and across systems.

CHANGE AND VALUES

The earliest philosophers theorized about change and its relationship to reality. Heraclitus believed reality to be "a continuous process of change and becoming, a world of dynamic stresses, of creative tensions between opposites"(9). For Parmenides, reality is a "solid, uncreated, eternal, motionless, changeless, uniform shape"(9, p. 60). Plato equated change with degeneration. These views of change are still very evident today, especially in the nursing system, where the pull between social traditions and scientific progress is often strong.

For example, nursing departments in certain hospital systems seem untouched by time. Strict dress codes and submission to authority are not questioned. There is a large core of nurses who have been practicing in the institution for many years. New ideas and new ways of thinking are discouraged because "we've always done things this way." Experimentation with new nursing roles is rare. There is a strong sense of tradition and adherence to many rules and rituals associated with that tradition. There may be an elaborate bureaucracy as in the military or civil service health care settings. One might describe such a nursing department as having a Platonic view of change.

At the other extreme are nursing departments within hospital systems that are in constant change. There is little uniformity in the way nurses dress as long as they are identifiable to patients. People working in clinical supervisory capacities are viewed more as consultants and resource persons than as bosses or authority figures. There is a steady flow of communication between the nursing staff and other professionals in the hospital. Conflict is dealt with openly, and often formal lines of communication are bypassed. The most dominant tradition is one of experimentation and innovation particularly with models of care delivery.

Consumer/clients in both hospitals may be satisfied with the care. However, nurses in the first work environment might consider the second type disorganized, and nurses from the second type of hospital might consider the first anachronistic. The first group of nurses highly values permanence and stability; the second group values constant change and movement.

KOAN

How do you value change? Does your value system permit a balance of stability and a willingness to change? For a self-assessment of how you perceive and grapple with change, answer these questions:

1. Do I concentrate more on defining the questions or on projecting the solutions in the change process?

2. Do I believe that rapid change is deleterious?
3. Do I overemphasize permanence and order?
4. Am I willing to entertain ideas contradictory to my own?
5. Do I secretly believe my plan is the answer to the problem?
6. Can I view the change from another person's point of view? Another system's point of view?
7. How many changes have occurred recently in my life? In my job?
8. Is there a pattern or pace to change in my experience?

In considering a specific change problem:

9. Can I change my premise from positive to negative and examine it?
10. Can I arrange my plan for change in sequential order, change the sequence, and contemplate the effects?
11. Can I isolate the critical factor in my change problem?
12. Can I consider my change within an historical time frame?
13. Can I project the effect of this change on the total system?

A MODEL OF CHANGE

There are many models and concepts proposed in attempts to understand and control the processes of change.

Watzlawick, Weakland, and Frisch have formulated a conceptual framework for understanding the phenomena of change within systems(10). Their theory is rooted in mathematical logic and is concerned with the peculiar interdependence of change and persistence and with system changes across boundaries and between hierarchical levels. "The tendency has been either to view persistence and invariance as a 'natural' or 'spontaneous' state, to be taken for granted and needing no explanation, and change as the problem to be explained, to take the inverse position"(10, p. 2). A brief description of the two types of change postulated (see below) may lead us to believe that second-order change is what nursing is in need of, but first-order change is what nurses generally initiate to manage problems and perpetuate persistence.

Type of Change	Definition[a]
First-order change	Change that occurs within a system with the system itself remaining essentially unchanged. There is no change in the basic rules or structure of the system, merely a rearrangement or manipulation of a part or parts of the system.
	1. Appears to be based on common sense
	2. Asks the question "why"
	3. Addresses itself to causes
	4. Is usually based on precedent or a "more of the same" recipe
Second-order change	Change of change. It is an occurrence that changes the system itself. It provides a way out of the original system. It changes the rules and internal order of the structure thus changing the system itself.
	1. Often appears wierd, illogical, unexpected, puzzling
	2. Is action oriented instead of origin oriented
	3. Solutions are dealt with
	4. Solutions are dealt with in the here and now
	5. Change techniques deal with effects not causes
	6. Crucial question is "what" not "why"

[a] The definitions of change were extracted from Watzlawick, Weakland, and Frisch (10).

There is no greater value to be attached to either type of change. Both can be used effectively or ineffectively, as in the case of the Carlucci family and staff-family communication, described on page 118.

The Carlucci family huddled in the tiny waiting area outside the Coronary Care Unit, anticipating news of their family member John, who had suffered a massive coronary myocardial infarction. John was 42 years old, a father of two sons, and a construction worker who also supported his widowed mother and youngest brother Joe, who was attending college.

The family had been waiting for an hour without information. John's mother and wife sat in a corner clutching one another. His brother paced. Repeatedly, Joe approached nurses and doctors who entered and left the unit. He was told to "wait, someone would be out shortly." Finally Joe angrily threatened to barge into the CCU if he could not get the information he needed.

No information was forthcoming. Joe rushed through the CCU doors, pushed aside protesting nurses and technicians, and went to his brother's bedside. He became very frightened when he saw his brother lying sedated, pale, and attached to several machines and tubes. When the security guards came to the unit to ask him to leave, Joe became agitated and resisted their intervention. A brief physical scuffle developed in view of most of the patients. Finally Joe was evicted, and the nursing care coordinator came to calm the staff and patients. The next day, at an emergency meeting of the ICU/CCU committee, the members, at the urging of the nursing staff, unanimously approved a motion to move the family waiting room from outside the ICU/CCU to a room off the main lobby of the hospital, two floors below. Administration agreed with the new policy and acted promptly to effect the change.

The fundamental problem of the inadequacy of communication between staff and families was not addressed or resolved in any way. The rules and the internal order of the communication system between family and staff were not changed. Only one very concrete component of the communication system was shifted— the location of the waiting room. This solution would probably lead to a new set of more serious problems, since the physical distance between patients and family members was increased. This is a classic example of *first-order change* that rearranges components of the system while insuring its structural and operational persistence.

Nurse groups invest vast amounts of energy and time in discussing and effecting first-order changes. Opposing factions within a nurse group engaged in problem solving often bring about first-order changes that, in fact, change nothing at all.

The first graduating class of a program leading to an associate degree in nursing asked the faculty to sponsor a capping ceremony as the culmination of their educational experience. This request precipitated a philosophical debate among faculty members. Four basic positions were presented: *(1)* **The cap is an important symbol in nursing, and the ceremony should be held because symbolism is so important to the late adolescent and tradition should be respected.** *(2)* **The capping ceremony should not be held, since the cap is inextricably connected with diploma school education.** *(3)* **A pinning ceremony would be a reasonable alternative, since other collegiate programs have held pinning ceremonies.** *(4)* **No special ceremony should be sponsored by the nursing department because such a ceremony would emphasize the differences between nursing and other college disciplines at a time when nursing was trying to gain legitimacy in the academic setting.**

Each position was eloquently defended by its supporters. When the vote was called, the compromise position, a pinning ceremony, was accepted, and the faculty endorsed and sponsored a pinning ceremony.

Switching from capping to pinning is certainly a first-order change, since the custom of performing a ritual or a rite of passage unique to nursing continues. What is the value to the individual nurse and to the nursing profession of switching from capping to pinning? Is not the traditional academic graduation ceremony at the culmination of a program sufficient to legitimize the completion of a nursing program within an academic community? Nursing is ambivalent in matters of tradition and attempts to deal with its ambivalence through first order change techniques.

KOAN

What is the value and function of ritual and symbolism to the nursing system? Has the nursing system used its rituals and symbols to change or to stay the same?

Second-order changes in the nursing system have been few, which is understandable, since the modern nursing system is still very young. It is a little over 100 years since Nightingale effected many major changes in the disorganized and amorphous nursing and health care systems of the late 1800s by using second-order change strategies. Three such second-order changes were (1) the formalization of nursing education; (2) the revamping of the structure and function of hospitals; and (3) the legitimization of the nursing profession as a means of employment for respectable women. Nightingale, who was to the end a proper upper-class gentlewoman, certainly must have appeared weird and illogical in her goals and strategies to her Victorian contemporaries. She dealt with solutions in the here and now. Using the political process and arousing public support through the newspapers were change techniques frequently employed by Nightingale. Her strategies were action oriented and did not necessarily rehash the causes of how things got that way, although there is no doubt that Nightingale knew her history. Finally, Nightingale focused on the whats and not on the whys in her attempts to change the system.

It is simpler to illustrate second-order changes by considering smaller social systems–dyadic or small-group systems, or subsystems within a larger system such as a hospital.

An experienced, intelligent registered nurse returned to college as a candidate in a baccalaureate degree program. She began having difficulty with a nursing instructor who was rather open in her disapproval of the student's independence and assertiveness. The instructor missed few opportunities to catch the student in minor errors in technique and to expose the student's shortcomings to her peer

group. The registered nurse student was so irritated by this that she tended to use even more independent and challenging behaviors, to which the instructor responded with more criticism. The situation escalated as the semester progressed. The registered nurse student considered dropping out of the program before the instructor failed her.

The nurse student discussed her dilemma with a friend, a clinical specialist in mental health nursing, who was on the faculty. The clinical specialist gave her friend a behavior prescription to follow. She instructed the registered nurse student to change from wearing her regular white nurse's uniform on clinical lab days to the blue student uniform of the school of nursing. (Registered nurse students were not required to buy the student uniforms of the college.) If the instructor questioned her new garb she was to say, "I'm really getting into the student role," and then move quickly out of the situation, before the instructor could reply.

At first the nursing student was appalled by the idea. "I could never bring myself to go back to the student uniform!" she retorted. After some thought she found the idea amusing and viewed the situation with great anticipation. She borrowed a student uniform from a friend and wore it on the next clinical day. The instructor never questioned the change but was helpful, kind, and rather pleasant to her. They got along well after that day.

Second-order change tactics can be quite effective and long lasting in dyadic systems. Watzlawick might theorize that in this situation nothing had really changed between the two parties.

Looking at a situation from a different perspective is often an effective form of problem solving, since the threatening situation that was once viewed as a vicious circle can be viewed differently. Reframing the problem creates flexibility in thinking and promotes the realization that one can deal differently with the problem situation. "This then brings about a change in one's behavior which is transmitted through the multiple and very subtle channels of human communication which affects the interpersonal reality in the desired form, even if the actual behavior prescription is never resorted to"(10, p. 131). The registered nurse student in the situation just described learned through experience that one way of guaranteeing change in a system is to *change oneself first.* Other changes must follow as the system shifts and adapts to any change.

Second-order change within larger nursing systems can be illustrated by the following example.

The director of nursing at a community hospital was concerned about unit 4 South. There was a high turnover of personnel in the unit and a higher number of incident reports than from any other nursing unit in the hospital. In addition, complaints from patients about uninterested nurses on 4 South were frequent. In a concentrated effort to deal with these problems, the director arranged for the head nurse to take a management course at the local university. She directed the supervisor of the unit to meet with the staff on a weekly basis in an effort to determine why the present system was not working well. She hired two more nurses for the unit and worked with the director of staff development to plan a six-month inservice program dealing with the nurse's responsibilities to the patient and the employer. Six months later, incident reports, complaints, and staff turnover remained high. Exasperated, the director met with a nurse consultant knowledgeable in change theories. The consultant pointed out to the director that all the changes instituted were first order, and while some of them worked for a while, the system itself remained basically unchanged. The staff, the consultant, and the director established an action plan for second-order change that included implementation of a nursing care delivery system that shifted the focus of accountability from supervisor to patient and that placed the nurses in the position of consultants to patients and families rather than of custodians and caretakers. The mobility of nurses increased as they were encouraged to make home visits to ensure continuity of care through effective discharge planning. The changes instituted represented a shift from the traditional model of caregiving to the primary model, which entailed changes in the rules, structure, and internal order of this nursing subsystem.

Large-scale nursing systems such as hospital nursing departments are likely to be complex and difficult to explore and influence. However, the basic principles of first- and second-order change can be applied in analyzing the "common problems, impasses, escalations and grand programs that are structurally identical to those encountered in the more personal areas of human life"(10, p. 158). An analysis of a nursing system that changed will serve as an illustration.

A CASE OF CHANGE IN A NURSING SYSTEM*

After a year of escalating conflict among nursing administration, medical administration, and hospital administration in a medium-sized community hospital, the following events occurred:

On a January evening in 1975 the administrator of the community general hospital dismissed the director of nursing and the associate administrator. The administrator took this action because of the director's alleged "unwillingness to communicate and cooperate with other departments." Members of the nursing staff who had been aware of administrative tensions for some time spontaneously formed picket lines outside the hospital. Some carried signs bearing messages such as "Medical Imperialism Wins Again," "Nurse Patients, Not Doctors," and "Doctors Are Not Gods." The placards succinctly captioned the issues. Who manages the department of nursing? To whom is the professional nurse accountable for her practice? To the patient, the physician, or the administration? These nurses took a risk in their decision to object to the actions of the hospital administration and the medical department. The protest was based strictly on the principle of the professional nurse's right to practice nursing. The nurses felt that both the medical and hospital administration had repeatedly interfered in their rights to practice professional nursing and to manage the practice of professional nursing. They took their case to the public.

This incident, which took place at St. Agnes Hospital in Philadelphia, Pennsylvania, was the culmination of the evolution of a nursing department within the hospital system over a 2½-year

*All excerpts in italics on the following pages are reprinted with permission from Donnelly, Mengel, and King(11).

span. It is not unusual for a director of nursing who has been progressive in practice and education and supportive of the nurse's right to practice as a semiautonomous professional to be dismissed when other parts of the administrative triad are upset by the imbalances in this delicate triangle (Fig. 4-2) caused by a change in one part.

A strikingly similar situation occurred in Lincoln, Nebraska, at Lincoln General Hospital, where the director of nursing was fired for alleged uncooperativeness with others in the hospital system who remained unidentified. The director of nursing had the support of the nursing staff at Lincoln General as well as the published support of the Nebraska Nurses Association. The director of nursing claimed that during her tenure, areas of responsibility and authority for nurses were clearly delineated and non-nursing duties that increase hospital costs and lessen the quality of service to patients were eliminated. "Anything which diverts the nurse's focus from the patient must be resolved, even the physician who insists that the nurse see that he has an ashtray at his elbow at all times," the director of nursing was quoted as saying in the *Lincoln Nebraska Journal,* December 19, 1971, p. 11. Her efforts to clarify and support nursing's role and to *collaborate* with the medical department led directly to her dismissal. Firing a strong director of nursing is certainly one way of keeping a nursing department weak and in a state of confusion.

In Dallas, Texas, at St. Paul's Hospital, another director of nursing was dismissed for asserting the professional rights of the nursing staff. The majority of the hospital's nursing staff wore black armbands at work in protest and demanded an investigation of the dismissal by the hospital's board of directors and the Daughters of Charity, who owned the hospital. The nurses claimed that the director of nursing was fired because of her open support of the revised Texas Nurse Practice Act, which was in legislative committee at the time of the dismissal. The Texas Nurse Practice Act, which by 1977 had not been revised for 53

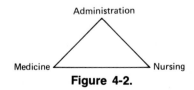

Figure 4-2.

years, permitted "unlicensed persons to function within hospitals in areas in which they aren't qualified and which endanger all of us in need of health care," a spokesperson for the nurses was quoted as saying in the *Dallas Morning News*. Despite opposition to the act from the Texas Hospital Association and the administration of St. Paul's Hospital, the director of nursing openly supported the new act and lost her job. This seemed to be a clear message to members of the nursing staff who remained and to other directors of nursing in Texas.

KOAN

If you were a staff nurse working in either of the two institutions in the above cases what would have been your response to the firing of the nursing directors?

What concerns would you have for your own position in the hospital system?

Would you have made your opposition or approval of the firings open and public? Why?

No doubt there are many similar incidents that have gone unrecorded and have ended in quiet defeat. The issues in these situations relate to control and to the establishment of a well-defined territory for nursing. In each case it appeared that as soon as the nursing department moved toward a clearer delineation of its purpose, other systems in the hospital responded vigorously. Medicine responds to keep its control over decision-making in patient care and over the nurse as "handmaiden." Administration responds to keep control of the nurse as employee. Corwin and Taves have observed that "the drive to gain professional status and achieve a unique place of importance within the hospital's division of labor inevitably brings the group [nurses] into conflict with the lay administration and physicians who are jealous of their prima donna status within the hospital scheme"(12). So, just as Sisyphus approached the top of the hill in Philadelphia, Lincoln, and Dallas, the gods became angry and the stone rolled down again.

Levenstein asserts that any change in a system that may alter one's status in the social structure may produce resistance from within the system. For example, when the hypodermic needle was made available, physicians debated whether to permit nurses to administer them lest the "time-honored dignity of the medical profession be impaired"(13). Physicians guard their power and status in the system jealousy. Nurses are increasingly seeking power and status in the system so that they can accomplish goals and provide a higher quality of service in response to consumer needs.

St. Agnes had the type of nursing department that a member of the board termed "a monster—too bright, too well educated, and too well functioning" for a community hospital. A professional performance committee, with representation from all levels of professional nursing, defined standards, evaluated the quality of care, and made recommendations for change. Job descriptions were based on the new Pennsylvania Nurse Practice Act and ANA Standards of Practice. Continuing education and staff development were recognized as essential to clinical competence and to professional development. Furthermore, a very close relationship existed between practice and education. Several nurses in the practice department held joint appointments in the school of nursing, and members of each group served on all nursing committees.

The nurses at this institution evolved from the type of nurse who was part of the hospital family, followed doctor's orders, and was loyal to the institution into the type of nurse who questions, thinks, and extends loyalty beyond the institution to the client and to a larger professional and social commitment. Physicians have traditionally given primary allegiance to their professional status rather than to organizational status. This commitment to professional status is increasing among nurses, even though they are employees rather than free entrepreneurs. Among many of the nurses at St. Agnes Hospital in Philadelphia, loyalty to the goals of their profession superseded allegiance to the institution. These are only a few of the indications that the potential for institutional conflict may increase in the future.

Ewing cites several other reasons for the breakdown of absolute loyalty and obedience to the employer that has been occurring in service institutions and industry. The first is young people's consciousness of rights that has been raised by the movements to establish the rights of women, minority groups, prisoners, and hospital patients. Young people educated in the recent more permissive atmospheres in colleges and universities find it difficult to work in organizations in which "all the rights (except for equal opportunity, safety, and labor law constraints) belong to the employer"(14). This certainly was true of many of the protesting nurses at Saint Agnes Hospital. Traditionally nurses have been loyal employees working in hospitals that may have subsidized their training. The emphasis was on responsibility and loyalty to the institution. Moving nursing education into colleges and universities has ultimately affected the delicate balance of power and control in hospital systems.

The second reason for the breakdown of absolute employee loyalty is increased worker participation in determining company policy in areas relating to job methods, work arrangements, and hours of work. The nursing staffs in many institutions are encouraged to participate in this type of policy formulation within the department of nursing, through committee participation, the setting of standards, and nursing care evaluation procedures.

The politicization of the corporation is the third reason contributing to the erosion of employee loyalty. "No longer do most Americans think of companies as private property which owners can manage as they please. Instead, companies are seen as public services, accountable to employees and consumers as well as to their stock holders"(14, p. 58). Hospitals are clearly accountable to the immediate community they serve and to larger society. If employees have good reason to oppose administrative rulings, and administration uses oppressive tactics in retaliation, is not administration shirking its responsibility both to its employees and to society?

Ewing believes that these trends will produce even more questions about the rights of all employees, with "limited rights to free speech, free press and privacy being targets of attention. It is likely that some leading companies will formulate and announce such rights voluntarily; others will wait until the law, unions, and employee associations or public pressure force them to grant certain rights"(14, p. 59). Had the three hospital administrations discussed been more sensitive to these trends the outcome of the incidents might have been very different.

The democratization of the nursing department and the increasingly high visibility of members of the management team were factors that contributed to the increased rate of change in the nursing system at St. Agnes Hospital.

Weekly nursing rounds were made by top nursing management personnel in an effort to provide a visible and accessible nursing management team. Rounds were conducted to reinforce the philosophy that a manager helps the provider deliver quality nursing care. The role of the nursing care coordinators and the clinical nursing specialists was to be supportive resource people and role models for the staff. The department of nursing concentrated on developing a cohesive staff with a philosophy that nursing is patient care and nurses are independent practitioners who should be skilled, accessible, and accountable to the patient for nursing care.

The nursing administration at St. Agnes Hospital began to explore management structures that were not vertically hierarchical in design (see Chap. 1). The nursing administration also planned a pilot project to demonstrate the efficacy of primary nursing care in one nursing unit where the nurses were eager to test the primary nursing system. Clinical specialists were employed to act as consultants to both patients and staff. The employment of these clinical specialists must certainly have been considered a second-order change to some physicians in the system.

The circumstances surrounding the arrival of the first psychiatric nursing clinical specialist was typical of the institution's resistance to second-order change. The clinical specialist interpreted her role as one of consultation initiated by other nurses or health professionals for the purpose of providing better nursing care through increased understanding of the patients' emotional responses to their illnesses. Some attending physicians and department heads objected to the fact that the clinical specialist did not report directly to a staff psychiatrist instead of to the director of nursing. Although some attending physicians and residents readily called upon the specialist about the emotional well-being of the patients, there was an almost equal number who told nurses that they did not want her to see or consult about their patients. This created an serious dilemma. Should the physicians' demands be honored even at the expense of denying patients the nursing care to which they are entitled? Or should the demands be ignored, again forcing the issue into open conflict? Should the psychiatric nursing clinical specialist insist upon access to the patient and the freedom to practice within the scope of her professional and legal rights and responsibilities?

Controversy surrounding the role of the psychiatric nurse clinician can be classified as a territorial skirmish. Certain physicians were upset at the idea of a nurse clinician seeing their patients without a written physician's order. The question arose again: Who has jurisdiction in decision-making for patient care? With whom does a patient contract for care once he or she is admitted to a hospital—the hospital, with its full range of services, including specialized nursing programs, or with the physician alone?

During the California nurses' strike of 1974, physicians were concerned that their control over patients would erode. Bradford Cohn, M.D., then president of the San Francisco Medical Society said, "I do not feel the hospital has any right, and it has no capacity, of entering into an agreement with CNA (California Nurses Association) that would abrogate the physician's rights and obligations toward patients. We, as physicians, have the deepest respect for all of our colleagues in the health care field. . . . This is especially true of registered nurses. . . . However, we must make it abundantly clear that the physician, and only the physician, has entered into a binding contact with *his* patient which makes him legally, ethically, and morally responsible for complete and total supervision and management of that patient's medical care"(15).

As the care of hospitalized patients proceeds on a day-to-day basis, territories and boundaries between medicine and nursing often blur, and neither profession strongly objects. However, in a power struggle, viewpoints comparable to the one voiced by the former president of the San Francisco Medical Society are advanced by most of the physicians involved. It is interesting to note the resurrection of Hippocrates each time physicians' domination of the health care system is threatened. No doubt there will be many more battles over the issues of territories and role boundaries before nurses' positions are well established in the health care delivery system.

It was a small group of physicians (not more than 10) [at St. Agnes Hospital] who repeatedly interfered in the administration of the nursing department and lodged complaints concerning the quality of care. Five of these physicians held administrative posts within the Department of Medical Affairs. Most of the attending staff were either uninvolved or on the fringes of the controversy when it erupted. The physicians in administrative positions had strong cultural and professional ties with each other. They seemed baffled by independent, thinking women and uncertain of their relationships with them. They found their relationships with the men nurses even more awkward. When they found themselves in a conflict situation with nurses, the physicians frequently invoked the "Captain-of-the-Ship" theory to defend their interference in nursing affairs. At one point, one department head physician demanded that a nursing care coordinator be removed from "his" area because he could not work with her. When nursing management refused to move the coordinator, the physician enlisted the aid of the administrator who yielded to his demand for the "good of the institution." Nursing management was shocked and disheartened at this administrative capitulation and interference. When the same physician experienced difficulty relating to the new coordinator appointed by the administrator, tensions escalated between nursing and medicine. In mid-December, at a medical staff meeting, the same group of physicians lobbied for the resignation of the director of nursing. The motion, made by the chief of surgery and seconded by the chief of medicine, was carried. It was a brief meeting with two items on the agenda: the dismissal of the director of nursing and the problem with inadequate space in the doctor's parking lot.

Although only a small fraction of the medical staff was vocal in their opposition to the changes in nursing practice and administration instituted by the nursing department, this small group became the ruling minority because of the abstention and lack of involvement of the silent majority, among the medical staff. Those most threatened by the redefinition of male-female roles as an outgrowth of the women's and nurses' rights movement, responded defensively by invoking the Captain-of-the-Ship argument (see Chap. 3).

The captain-of-the-ship theory, though frequently invoked by doctors, has been successfully challenged in the courts. It holds only in very special circumstances(see Chap. 3.)

In every state in the country, a nurse is legally liable for her actions even if she is following a doctor's order. Nurses can and have been sued in such cases(14, p. 58).

In principle, the physician who demands that a nurse be removed from "his" unit is no different from the physician ordering that a nurse give an improper dosage of medication. This is a classic example of what Veatch classifies as the generalization of expertise syndrome(16). Generalization of expertise can be defined as a condition that arises "when, consciously or unconsciously, it is assumed that an individual with scientific expertise in a particular area also has expertise in the value judgments necessary to make policy recommendations simply because he has scientific expertise(16). The physician is prone to believe that he has "special moral requirements which do not extend to the general public . . ." including nurses and other health professionals(16). Thus when a physician demands that a nurse give a medication that the nurse believes to be unsafe, a physician may react negatively to the refusal because his expertise has been questioned. Physicians often make choices for patients and their families without exploring the alternatives. For example, how often is the sick person given the choice of what hospital to go to? How often are hospital patients informed of the range of services available to which they have a right? How often are alternative approaches to a health problem explored with patients and their families?

The firing of the director of nursing at St. Agnes Hospital may well have been the result of too many open challenges to the generalized expertise of a few physicians in the system. Following the firing of the director of nursing at the Philadelphia hospital,

. . . certain attending physicians and residents became increasingly intimidating to nurses. One physician threatened to "fire" a nurse for questioning a medication order. Another physician would not explain his rationale for an unusual medication order. When questioned by the nurse concerning this order, he replied flippantly, "It's a secret." The director of the school of nursing

was accused of including "disrespect to physicians" in the curriculum. By the end of December relationships between the nursing and medical departments had sharply deteriorated.

After the dismissal of the top nursing administration, nursing personnel chose resignation as a final form of protest. One-half of the faculty of the school of nursing, two clinical specialists, five nursing care coordinators, the president of the Staff Nurses Association, several head nurses, the director of the school of nursing, the director of nursing practice, and several staff nurses resigned. From a staff of approximately 140 professional nurses, 33 resigned.

In their book, Weisband and Frank enumerate four choices that government officials who have reached a crisis of conscience in their jobs should explore before taking action. These same four choices may be considered as alternatives by many nurses who face a crisis of conscience(17).

1. They can stay on the job quietly, hope for the best, and try to resist the system covertly from the inside.
2. They can exit quietly and sever their connection with "the team."
3. They can leave with public protest and alert the public to the dangers in the system or the policy with which they disagree.
4. They may try to have it both ways and hold the job for as long as possible, then exit because they are torn between remaining discreetly silent and protesting publicly.

Weisband and Frank believe that most people in high-level positions in the executive branch of the United States government choose the second option. The practice of leaving silently has probably been the predominant option chosen by nurses as well. However, the nurses in St. Agnes Hospital situation chose to leave in large numbers and with public protest. Subsequently, many had difficulty finding new positions. Many, for a time, were disillusioned with nursing's lot in the health care system. But all of them survived the experience and learned from it.

> ## KOAN
>
> What is the cost of silence? What is the price of protest?

Men and women in positions of power and responsibility who choose not to pay the price of personal integrity merely succeed in shifting those costs to society as a whole. America . . . has been paying the price of a political tradition that fosters conformity rather than conviction and group loyalty rather than individual accountability, that borrows its terminology from the language of corporate athletics—in which a man's willingness to "play ball" is his true measure—rather than from moral ethics(17, p. 1).

Reflections on a Case of Change

In the St. Agnes case, the hospital system initially adjusted easily to first-order changes introduced by the nursing department. In fact, the hospital administration provided the nursing department with positive feedback on the changes. Positive feedback tends to accelerate change in systems. Second-order changes exemplified by the addition of the nursing clinical specialists, detailed nursing research studies, and a collegial approach to physicians seemed too much for the system to bear.

Before the hiring of the director of nursing who was ultimately dismissed, St. Agnes Hospital's nursing department was well integrated into the traditionalism of the total hospital system. After approximately two years of both first- and second-order changes within the nursing department, the system imbalances emerged in the power struggles just described.

Did the nursing subsystem miscalculate the potential for second-order change? Did it misread the risks? Were the changes introduced in such a way that their acceptance was doomed? If the nurses could have predicted the outcome could they, should they, have stopped their course of action? Did the physicians misconstrue the changes? Or did they perceive them correctly and continue their concerted effort to block them? More likely, the changes did not fit their concept of the known. Physicians are a vested-interest group who traditionally have great authority and power. Why relinquish it for nursing's avowed patient-advocate orientation? Such professed humanitarian values certainly must seem foreign to some physicians in the real world of the hospital. Others, less trusting, often interpret the advocate position as an inarguable means of nurses gaining power. With challenges to their authority from consumers, the media, the government, and nurses, physicians appear to be reacting in an understandably defensive manner. They have consciously or subconsciously decided to fight the nearest and most intimate group they know—nursing—which may also be the weakest group because it is so easily splintered and because new nurses are so easily recruited to replace the dissenters. The law of supply and demand has often worked against the advancement of nursing.

Eric Hoffer contends that revolution most often occurs after a major change(18) or, in terms of Watzlawick *et al.*, after a second-order change(10). By introducing into the system at St. Agnes Hospital enough nurses with an irreverence for past roles and relationships and with a strong determination to practice collegially with physicians, the nursing system instituted a second-order change, and the physicians revolted. The nurses at St. Agnes Hospital did not realize that they were following a natural evolutionary process. By looking at events from an historical perspective, one can often, although not always, predict the trends and outcomes. High-level nursing management had "turned over" at St. Agnes Hospital approximately every two years for the previous eight years. What remained constant in the hospital was the physician management system. The nursing system trusted the organizational chart to define interorganizational relationships operationally. In reality, the physician management system made the major decisions regarding the interorganizational roles and relationships.

After years of experience in exercising their substantial authority over government and insurance companies, physicians have become skillful political maneuverers. Nurses are still lacking in these skills for a number of reasons. One reason is that the AMA has long been a potent influence in the legislative process. Only recently has the ANA established a political action arm to demonstrate to its members the necessity for political skills and involvement.

In addition, there exists a high turnover rate in hospital nursing personnel and in nursing in general. This results in less investment by nurses in the politics of the work setting and the profession. In the past, when a nurse did not like the politics of an institution, a graceful exit was easy because of the number and variety of job opportunities. A tighter nursing job market in the future may change the easy exit solution. Furthermore, in the past nurses tended to think of themselves as not responsible for their own actions. Some nurses still operate under this assumption; that is, that the physician is the captain of the ship and that he and the hospital are responsible for the nurse's actions. Now that changing nurse practice laws and consumers hold nurses more strictly accountable for their actions, nurses are growing more knowledgable and are asking more questions of physicians. Such situations have created a proliferation of a previously rare species—the political nurse.

However, even the nurses in the St. Agnes case, despite their education and experience, were naive in reading and reacting to the political situation. In their zeal and naivete, the nurses assumed that, since they absolutely believed that their cause was good, right, and desirable, truth and justice would support their position. The situation as it evolved, however, confirms the fact that good intentions in trying to alter a system are virtually irrelevant, particularly for nurses who, unlike physicians, are paid employees. "The courts have made it clear that employees exercise the privilege of free speech at their own risk, however reasonable their motives"(14, p. 55). Nurses must keep in mind constantly that what they view as ethical may not necessarily be viewed that way by others in the health system.

It is easily forgotten that one group's values will inevitably conflict with another group's values. When this occurs the group with the greatest political skills and the most social and economic power will win, even though the total system may lose. Within the health care system, the climate seems ripe for second-order change. Nursing has the opportunity to be the impetus for many of these changes. However, the risk factor is high. It is certain that any change will spawn new sets of problems and demand new sets of behaviors. The process is continuous. The nursing system should adjust to the fact that it must travel hopefully and confidently and learn to influence the journey, because arriving at a final "destination" is a myth.

PLANNED CHANGE: IS IT REALLY POSSIBLE?

Management literature is replete with simplistic notions concerning planning and effecting change. Some of these guidelines reflect commonsense principles that came to light as members of organizations struggled with the change process. These simplistic guidelines, though sometimes helpful, are not always applicable to change in complex systems such as the health care system, the nursing system, and the hospital system. Table 4-1 contrasts simplistic notions for dealing with change with guidelines for dealing with change in complex systems. Try to apply this information to the changes that took place in the hospital systems and nursing subsystems that have been discussed so far.

Within a systems framework, the change process becomes more difficult to understand and to predict as the complexity of the system increases. The traditional problem-solving method—assessment, planning, implementation, evaluation—with its linear approach, often does not work as satisfactorily as might be hoped. For example, just as a nurse manager completes an assessment of a problem and draws up a plan, problem variables may change so that the plan devised is no longer totally relevant.

The phrase *planned change* is somewhat paradoxical, since change is the constant of any system. Traditional change theory portrays the system and the change as if the two were in some way in opposition. Low explains that in monolithic organizations such as hospitals, it is often felt that the system acquires significance by remaining stable(19). Hierarchical structuring, with its tendency toward power structuring, enables systems to become inert or to resist change. Although inertia provides stability in the system, it also can inhibit the generation of new ideas and plans.

A change process that will not result in cataclysm and reorganization as in the St. Agnes incident requires a balance between stability, or stasis, and change (Fig. 4-3).

Table 4-1. A Comparison of Simplistic and Complexity-Oriented Guidelines for Dealing With Change in Systems

Simplistic Guidelines	Complexity-Oriented Guidelines
Change is more likely if persons affected by it have had a part in shaping it	Change in a system is a rule; it occurs constantly
If proposed changes are understood, their acceptance is more likely	Change is process; not content
Change that is systematically planned is more acceptable than haphazard change	Change begets change
Change that does not threaten the security of any one group is more acceptable	Every change has its price
Change is more likely when linked to a group's value system and beliefs	Change involves thinking, not merely rearranging prejudices
Change is acceptable if it follows a previously successful change rather than a change that failed	Change occurs according to a pattern or structure that may be unique to the system
Gradual change is more acceptable than sweeping change	Change may tend to accelerate systems
If people share in the benefits of change, acceptance is more likely	Change does not guarantee success

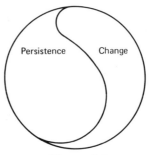

Persistence   Change

Figure 4-3.

Nurses are probably aware that systems change in many directions simultaneously: laterally, horizontally, and vertically. For example, as a nursing system (a department, a unit, the whole profession) exists, "its functions become increasingly more differentiated and complex (the lateral dimension). New systems, procedures and understandings bring about new integrations or a new orientation, and there is a tendency toward different and new wholes to be created . . . (the horizontal dimension. . . . As the [system] grows, higher level ideas are introduced enabling it to encompass an increasing field of phenomena (the vertical dimension)"(19, p. 3). In other words, to change only one part of a system is like trying to bake only half a cake. A total-system view will lead nurses to the realization that major changes in the nursing system inevitably will bring about changes in the larger health care system. Thinking about the change process, exploring alternatives for the future, selecting more than one possible course of action, and monitoring the effects of change on related systems will give nurses an advantage as they continue to struggle with and within changing systems.

KOAN

Is planned change in the nursing system really possible?
Is change best planned in learning environments?

REFERENCES

1. Nightingale F: *Notes on Nursing: What It Is, And What It Is Not.* Philadelphia, JB Lippincott Company, 1946.

2. Toffler A: *Future Shock.* New York, Random House, 1970, p 21.

3. Toynbee A: *Mankind and Mother Earth.* New York, Oxford University Press, 1976, p 590.

4. Reiser SJ: *Medicine and the Reign of Technology.* London, Cambridge University Press, 1978, p 166.

5. Buckley W: Society as a complex adaptive system in Buckley W (ed): *Modern Systems Research for the Behavioral Scientist.* Chicago, Aldine Publishing Company, 1968, p 493.

6. Toynbee A: *Civilization on Trial and The World and The West.* New York, World Publishing, 1971, p 45.

7. Dock L: Self Protrait. *Nurs Outlook* 25:22–26, 1977.

8. Styles M: Continuing education in nursing: One hope for professional coherence. *Nurse Educ* July-August, vol 1: 6–9, 1976.

9. Koestler A: *The Sleepwalkers.* London, Hutchinson and Company Ltd, 1959, p 60.

10. Watzlawick P, Weakland J, Fisch R: *Change.* New York, WW Norton & Co Inc, 1974.

11. Donnelly G, Mengel A, King E: Anatomy of a conflict. *Superv Nurse,* 6:28–38, 1975.

12. Corwin RG, Taves MJ: Nursing and other health professions cited by Schulz R, Johnson AC: Conflict in hospitals, in Levy S, Loomba NP (eds): *Health Care Administration.* Philadelphia, JB Lippincott Company, 1973, p 259.

13. Levenstein A: Effective change requires change agent. *Hospitals* 50: 71–74, 1974.

14. Ewing DW: Employee rights: Taking the gag off. *The Civil Liberties Review,* Fall, 1974, pp 54–61.

15. Phillips D: San Francisco nurses strike. *The Hospital Medical Staff,* October, 1974, pp 13–20.

16. Veatch RM: Generalization of expertise. *The Hastings Center Studies* 1:29–40, 1973.

17. Weisband E, Frank T: *Resignation in Protest: Political and Ethical Choices: Between Loyalty to Team and Loyalty to Conscience in American Public Life.* New York, Grossman, Publishers—a division of Viking Press, 1975, p 55.

18. Hoffer E: *The Ordeal of Change.* New York, Harper & Row Publishers Inc, 1963.

19. Low A: *Zen and Creative Management.* New York, Anchor Books, 1976, p 3.

CHAPTER **FIVE**
The Learning System

This is a critical period in nursing education and we must see clearly and build wisely if our work is to stand for the future. The first essential is that we should clear the ground of the old outworn or unsound timbers which are giving way under the strain of modern demands and the spirit of a new age. . . . If we have faith in our work and the world's need of it, we shall not fail.

*Isabel M. Stewart**

LEARNING AND PURPOSE

Isabel M. Stewart, a well-known nursing educator at Teachers College, Columbia University, delivered the message quoted above at a meeting in Boston in June 1921(1). The message could easily have been written today by someone surveying the current state of the nursing learning system. There is still great confusion and controversy over how and where nurses should be educated. The great nursing education debate and the ongoing efforts of nursing leaders to bring nursing into the mainstream of higher education continues unabated, more than a century after the establishment of the first schools of nursing in the United States.

*From reference 4.

141

Why has the nursing system supported so much diversity in its learning system? Would the adoption of a standard postgraduate curriculum like those in medicine and law have been more advantageous to both clients and to nurses? What are the advantages and disadvantages to a learning system that has several different educational settings, formats, and time requirements, including hospital programs, associate degree programs, and baccalaureate programs for preparing its beginning practitioners. While filling in Table 5-1, think about this question and formulate some conclusions. Read each statement of purpose carefully and discuss and reflect on which course of study and in which educational setting education toward the purpose could best be accomplished.

The learning system in nursing clearly illustrates nursing's confusion over its central purpose. Currently there are four types of preservice programs that result in eligibility to take a nurse licensing examination. There are the hospital school of nursing program requiring from 24 to 36 months of study, the two-year associate degree program usually conducted at a community college, the four-year baccalaureate or "generic" program conducted at a college or university, and the practical nursing program that is usually conducted in schools of practical nursing and requires eight months to one year of study. The practical nurse takes a different license examination than the one for professional nurse licensure. The examination for professional nurse licensure is taken by graduates from the hospital school, the associate degree program, and the generic baccalaureate program. Masters degree and doctoral programs in nursing further complicate the nursing learning system. It appears that nursing has constructed the same hierarchical pattern in its learning system as in its practice system (Fig. 5-1).

The learning system pyramid is further complicated by the addition of nurse practitioners in certification programs and master's prepared clinicians, who are sometimes educated through preceptorships with physicians as preceptors (Fig. 5-2).

Nursing, like many other systems, gravitates toward a hierarchical structure. The way in which a system is structured is not always a result of choice. Meyer and Rowan point out that organizations, like professions, "deal with their environments at their boundaries and imitate environmental elements in their structures"(2). There are some institutional theories that define an organization or as a profession as a "dramatic enactment of the

Table 5–1. Speculations on How Learning Systems Can Fulfill the Purpose of Nursing

Nursing Leaders	Purpose of Nursing Is	Course of Study	Educational Setting
Florence Nightingale	To put the patients in the best condition for nature to act upon them		
Lavinia Dock and Isabel Stewart	To promote and conserve health and prevent disease, protect and care for people's social and physical environment, and care for the whole person—mind and body		
Dorothy Johnson	To assist patients in the maintenance or reestablishment of a moving state of equilibrium throughout the health change process		
Virginia Henderson	To assist people, sick or well, in the performance of those activities contributing to health or its recovery (or to peaceful death) that they would perform unaided if they had the necessary strength, will, or knowledge, and to do this in such a way as to help them gain independence as rapidly as possible		
Sister Madeleine Clemence	To help patients become "authentic persons" and to use their situation, the illness, for doing so		
Martha Rogers	To help people achieve their maximum health potential. Nursing's first line of defense is promotion of health and prevention of illness. Care of sick is resorted to when our first line of defense fails		

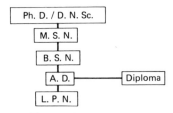

Figure 5-1.

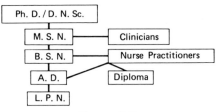

Figure 5-2.

rationalized myths pervading modern societies . . ." about that group(2, p. 346). What are the rationalized myths of modern society concerning nursing? Certainly the image of the nurse in the media (Chap. 1) is indicative of societal myth. Nursing, still predominantly a female occupation, is often presented as a group of nurturing, self-sacrificing, unobtrusive women who respond to and meet the needs of others. Roles and functions of nurses often change according to the institution's myths about the nurse. Even in the academic setting, the nursing faculty struggles to reconcile the myth of nursing and the values and demands of academia.

Is nursing's purpose so broad and amorphous that the system will continue to spawn new roles to fill the needs? A reexamination of Table 1-1, "Views on the Purpose of Nursing" directs the reader to consider each purpose of nursing and the course of study and educational setting that would most likely result in a fulfillment of that purpose. Is it possible to prepare the nurse to fulfill these broad purposes in a standardized program of nursing like the postgraduate curricula adopted by medicine and law? Can nursing reach beyond the rationalized myths of society and accomplish a sweeping reform in its learning system as medicine did in the early 1900s? Is the nursing system already in the midst of such reform?

NURSING AND MEDICINE LEARNING SYSTEMS: SOME PARALLELS

Currently in the United States there are few distinguished professional medical schools that are not connected to a university. "The trend has been to hold that good professional training is to be found only in the university professional school, where the faculty of the professional school in question is treated as part of a general university faculty"(3). Medicine traces its educational roots to the twelfth-century European universities, where the four standard faculties were theology, philosophy, law, and medicine. Medicine as we know it today, with its scientific, technological leanings may seem out of place among philosophy, theology, and law. However, historically, medicine's principle concerns were with the individual person and his or her biological ills. This focus on the individual fitted in well with the humanistic leanings of the early European universities.

In the Middle Ages, medicine as a scholarly discipline was taught only to master surgeons and physicians. The barber-surgeons, classified as tradesmen and guildsmen, practiced the hands-on crafts of medicine. The university-educated physicians controlled the barber-surgeons, who later freed themselves and established independent status with the right to a university education and degree(4). Control of groups such as midwives, apothecaries, barber-surgeons, and nurses, all of which the medical profession considered subordinate, has been an important issue in the medical profession since the Middle Ages. Stewart asserts that nursing's darkest period came during the Middle Ages, when medical science was renewing itself and when physicians were recouping their former prestige and power. The physician's "struggles with barber-surgeons, apothecaries, midwives, and other 'irregular' practitioners undoubtedly made him suspicious of all workers who might in any way threaten his economic security or his hard-won professional status"(4, pp. 24, 25). The themes of control and domination and separation and individuation are apparent to this day in the relationship between nursing and medicine, even though, through licensure, nursing had an opportunity to separate from medicine's control.

KOAN

Are nurse practitioners, nurse midwives, and other specially educated nurses posing the same threat to the medical profession as the barber-surgeons of the Middle Ages?

Medical education in America evolved quite differently from medical education in Europe. In the pre-Civil War era, medical education was conducted in proprietary schools. Proprietary schools were owned by a group of physicians and were business enterprises. The first privately owned proprietary medical college was owned and operated by three physicians and was set up at Castleton, Vermont in 1818(5). A prospective student would find, for a fee, a practicing physician to act as preceptor. The preceptorship was usually three years and consisted of practice along with two 3-month lecture courses.

> The lecture courses were ungraded and the second was identical to the first—tedium compounded. Earlier requirements for Latin and the M.D. thesis were by now defunct and since students were assessed a diploma fee, final examinations rarely took a scalp. Even the rule that medical graduates must be twenty-one was widely ignored(6).

Because of the growth in the number of proprietary schools after the Civil War too many physicians were produced. Many were of low quality, since academic standards tended to erode with so many schools competing for students. The American Medical Association (AMA) which was founded in 1847, became increasingly pessimistic about reform in the medical education system as the twentieth century approached. However, in the latter half of the 1800s the public school came into being, greatly expanding the opportunity for quality premedical education. At the turn of the

century there was a wide range of premedical education requirements. As early as 1893, Johns Hopkins University in Baltimore,
Maryland, required an academic degree before entrance into medical school. In contrast, the Council on Medical Education of the
American Medical Association in 1906 was still recommending a
minimum of one year of college for medical school admission(7).
This state of affairs illustrates how an individual institution or a
small group of creative individuals can often set a trend and a
standard more effectively than a large organization that represents many vested interests.

The trend in medical education in the late 1800s had been
toward higher standards. The AMA, however, had little effect on
reforming the system.

> Lacking any legal bite, the AMA sought to work by moral
> suasion alone. A main reason for it's failure is found in the
> structure of the AMA itself. . . . If physician-owners of prop-
> rietary schools were to be induced to join a national organi-
> zation which strongly favored educational reform, they
> would have to be offered greater voter representation than
> their numbers would dictate. On the other hand, of course,
> giving the medical schools too large a voice would block
> any chance for reform. . . . Perceiving that the AMA was
> essentially powerless, the physician-professors refused to
> participate and thus were free to ignore the AMA's exhorta-
> tions(6, p. 555).

Between 1890 and 1914, however, American medicine, largely
through the efforts of the AMA, moved toward professional matu-
rity. During this period medical societies, licensing associations,
and a leading group of colleges had common aims: "the upgrading
of entrance standards to the profession, the specification of curricula in the medical schools, the suppression of the weakest
proprietary institutions and the reduction in the number of students graduating from medical school"(8). The interlocking aims
of such reforms were partly educational—having more highly
educated practitioners—and partly economic—producing fewer
physicians, thus lessening competition.

The educational innovations at Johns Hopkins University,
which was modeled after the German university's research-

oriented medical schools, acted as a catalyst for reform of the medical education system. The use of science laboratories and hospital wards in the education of the physician and the establishment of full-time clinical professorships set standards that forced the closing of many of the weaker proprietary schools(8, p. 58). The Council on Medical Education of the AMA, formed in 1904, served, too, as a force in the reform of the medical education system. This council "periodically inspected medical schools and began a rating system of A (worthy), B, and C (hopeless). Their reports were broadcast and the ensuing publicity undoubtedly contributed to the closure or merger of twenty-nine schools between 1906 and Flexner's report four years later. . . . Dr. N. P. Colwell, secretary of the council, accompanied Flexner on several inspection trips and . . . his medical insights must have proved helpful to Flexner"(6, p. 545).

The impact of the Flexner report, which stands as a monument in the reform of medical education; was instrumental in finally shaping the medical education system that remains today. With the blessings and the assistance of the AMA, Flexner's meticulously documented report vividly described the poor conditions in the marginal schools and hastened their closing.

The American medical education system before 1910 was in a chaotic state. The public sensation caused by the Flexner report enabled the medical education system to purge itself by embarassing, weakening, and finally eliminating the marginal medical schools and to enlist financial support to accomplish reform. After the Flexner report was published in 1912, "John D. Rockefeller donated almost 50 million dollars to improve the nation's medical schools . . ."(6, p. 561).

Adoption of the standard four-year postgraduate curriculum as the minimum requirement in medical education accomplished not only the upgrading of standards and care but the equalizing of all physicians. "Once within the sheltered confines [of the profession] professional democracy was to reign"(8, p. 431).

This educational equality among members of the profession is something that nursing has never enjoyed. The evolution of the nursing learning system has been additive, that is, innovations such as the associate degree program were added to and grew out of existing nursing programs, unlike the medical system, whose reformers opened the door to a new and stable system. It could even be said that changes in the nursing learning system have been of a first-order nature (Chap. 4).

There are many parallels and differences that can be cited between the growth of the nursing and the medical education systems, at least up to the time of the Flexner report.

Unlike medicine, nursing has its educational roots in the Christian church, not in the university. The great monastaries of medieval Europe, with their absolute control over their members, provided a unique organizational structure for training groups of workers. In the monastic schools, nursing was not treated as an intellectual discipline with a body of knowledge. It was learned chiefly through practice and experience. Like agriculture, it was considered a manual art. Nursing also ranked high "as a form of spiritual discipline and was frequently prescribed as an antidote for moral diseases—pride, sloth, overfastidiousness, and the like. ... The special virtues in nursing as a medicine for sick souls were the hard physical work entailed and the often distasteful duties which were considered an effective means for mortifying the flesh and developing humility, patience and other Christian virtues"(4, p. 13).

Organized nursing evolved under both religious and military-like control from the Middle Ages well into the eighteenth century. Secular nurses (nurses not members of the religious nursing orders) were called servant nurses and received no formal training of any kind.

When Florence Nightingale began the massive reforms of the amorphous nursing system, nursing as an art was practiced on the one hand by lower-class poor women who drank and prostituted themselves and, on the other hand, by religious women who practiced nursing as part of their religious calling. Until Nightingale there was no middle ground. Although Nightingale believed nursing to be a calling or a vocation, she called for and engineered the secularization of the nursing profession. "Nursing now ceased to be a penance, a self-sacrifice, or a merit ensuring a high place in the next world, and was firmly established as an honorable, if laborious means of earning one's livelihood"(9).

With the sound economic underpinnings of the Nightingale fund (donated by the British public in gratitude for her war service) the Nightingale School began to prepare women not only to function in hospitals and infirmaries but to further reform nursing education and practice. Nightingale's aims were high. She carefully selected students and prepared them for leadership. Although she did not believe nursing to be a profession independent of medicine, she firmly held that a nurse was to work with a doctor but not be subservient to him as the lay servant nurses had been.

One of the most radical innovations of the Nightingale plan for the education of nurses was the recognition of science as a foundation for practice. From its inception, the Nightingale program included a heavy theoretical component as well as an experiential one. It was clear from the school's beginning that the probationers (beginning students) were indeed students, not merely helpers or domestics. The ward sisters (experienced nurses) who taught the students emphasized ways of observing and ways of thinking. Probationers were not overburdened with domestic chores or given premature responsibilities. Nightingale considered such practices economically unsound and wasteful of the potential of trained personnel. She once remarked, "A nurse should do nothing but nurse. If you want a charwoman, have one. Nursing is a specialty"(10).

KOAN

In settings where you have practiced and/or observed nursing, are nurses doing "nothing but" nursing? What percentage of the nurse's time is spent in nonnursing activities? How close is the model you are observing to Nightingale's concept of the nurse's role?

The Nightingale School embodied many of the characteristics of other areas of British education: *(1)* careful selection of students, *(2)* process-oriented instruction, *(3)* emphasis on the individual rather than the group, *(4)* practical work preceding formal instruction, and *(5)* supervised home life intended to act as a character-forming influence(4, p. 79).

The American version of the Nightingale plan was quick to capitalize on the new source of inexpensive labor that the hospital school of nursing could provide. Whereas the central purpose of the Nightingale school was to prepare nurses, the American schools emphasized other aims. Bellevue Hospital School of Nursing, for example, opened in 1873, published the following goals:

1. "To make this great Hospital a place where the respectable poor could be tenderly and skillfully nursed and where even . . . paupers would be sure of kindly and patient care."
2. "The training yearly of a band of *experienced, obedient, devoted nurses* for service in private cases or amongst the poor"(4, p. 11).

The original aims of the Bellevue school, patterned after the Nightingale model, and those to follow in the United States emphasized the service that could be rendered by the student nurses instead of the primacy of educating a specialist, a practitioner.

The organizational structure and economic underpinnings of the early American nursing schools are important in order to understand the present system and how it evolved. Economic and administrative decision-making in hospitals was largely dominated by physicians who, in many instances, were the founders of such hospitals. At the turn of the century, graduates, particularly from the Johns Hopkins Training School, were in demand to fill administrative and teaching positions in hospitals and to start schools of nursing. Nurse training schools were cost effective and even profit making for hospitals, since most of the care was provided by the steady stream of students through the school. An example of the profit potential of a nursing school was revealed in the 1878 report of a Hartford hospital that stated, ". . . pupil nurses had been sent out at the request of physicians throughout the state to care for 66 private cases during the year, the charge for their services being $10.00 per week and traveling expenses. School receipts, $1,948.83, exceeded disbursements by $1,097.69. Many other hospitals accepted the principle that the school must not only pay its way but must be an economic asset to the hospital"(4, p. 130).

In light of this, nursing leaders were often pressured to open training schools with few resources and little preparation. In the late 1890s one nursing leader of the period alleged "that when five doctors got together they started a hospital and that when they hired a day nurse and a night nurse they decided to hire a third nurse and make it a training school"(11).

By the turn of the century the number of hospitals was growing exponentially. In 1873 there were about 178 hospitals in the United States. By 1909 the number of hospitals had grown to 4,359 with a bed capacity of over 421,000. Nurse training schools also mushroomed during this period. Without the regulation of any formal body, hospitals took the initiative and gained control of existing schools and opened many others. In an address delivered to the New Jersey League of Nursing Education in 1928, Dr. George Hanlon pointed out that

> Hospitals very promptly recognized improved conditions in caring for the sick as the efficiency of the nursing school progressed. They were equally prompt to recognize the conspicuously low cost at which they secured nursing care and the obvious advantage to the hospital to have complete control of the schools. . . . In 1880 only 15 schools were integral parts of hospitals. In 1890 this had increased to thirty-five, by 1900 there were four hundred twenty-three, while today there are scarcely a dozen not so dependently linked(12).

The concomitant expansion of hospitals and nursing schools spawned a nursing education system that often exploited its students but at the same time engendered a loyalty to the training institution and its way of doing things. There was, however, wide divergence in the content and process of training programs. In fact, some programs were conducted on a correspondence basis. One such school, eventually driven out of business by the Pennsylvania State Board of Nursing, was the Philadelphia School for Nurses(13). This school, allegedly governed by several hundred physicians, advertised widely and offered various programs—one of 10 weeks duration and the other by correspondence. This school engaged in a bitter dispute with the State Board of Nurse Examiners over the board's refusal to grant its graduates registration. The school even petitioned the governor to dissolve the State Board of Nursing. The petition, of course, was not honored, and the school eventually closed. The bitterness of this case reflects nursing's struggle to gain control over its educational system, a struggle it still faces.

During this same period the medical education system, with the Flexner report as catalyst, was standardizing, upgrading, and streamlining its educational system. As medical education grew strong, the nursing system became more subject to medical domination and hospital control. Since the relationship between nursing and medicine has long been conceptualized along traditional male-female lines, organized medicine has always believed in its paternalistic right to speak out on questions of nursing education. Even though the Flexner report imposed rigorous educational requirements on the prospective physician, the notion of an educated nurse was met with great ambivalence by many.

As far back as the inception of the Nightingale School in England in 1860, prominent physicians who managed nurses under the old system at St. Thomas Hospital regarded the proposed Nightingale School as an affront. Dr. South, a senior surgeon at St. Thomas, wrote a pamphlet in opposition to the Nightingale School in which he declared that "the proposed school was quite unnecessary and superfluous . . ."(9, p. 179). His definition of the nurse's role reveals his traditional, classicist views. "As regards the nurses or wardmaids, these are in much the same position as housemaids and require little teaching beyond that of poultice-making, which is easily acquired, the enforcement of cleanliness, and attention to patients' wants"(9, p. 181).

Dr. La Garde, another contemporary of Nightingale, believed that communicating professional, technical knowledge to a nurse could be dangerous. "A nurse is a confidential servant but still only a servant. She should be middle-aged when she begins nursing; and if somewhat tamed by marriage and the troubles of a family so much the better"(9, p. 201).

Despite the vocal opposition of a few physicians, the indifference of the majority, and the support of a few, Nightingale's plan prevailed. In fact, Nightingale seems not to have wasted much energy worrying about what the opposition said or published. She asserted her own views and their rationale and persisted in enacting her plan. Perhaps Nightingale's secret was that she did not waste energy on reaction but conserved energy for action.

In the United States, too, in the late 1800s and early 1900s, the idea of educating nurses was met with some resistance by various groups. Physicians feared some loss of control and anticipated interference in matters of patient care that they viewed as their distinct domain. Hospital authorities were wary of educated nurses who might be "trouble makers and would not be willing to do the hard heavy work required in the hospital"(4, p. 89). As medicine assumed a dominant role in the education of nurses in the hospital schools and as hospital administrators realized the economic contribution of nursing students to the total hospital system, hospital schools flourished. In fact, there is a history of strong support of hospital school nursing programs by many medical subgroups and individuals that has persisted to the present.

In August 1928 at the nursing section of the American Hospital Association (AHA) meeting in San Francisco, the benefits of autonomous schools of nursing was discussed from various perspectives. Greener pointed out that in 1928 (nearly two decades after the publication of medicine's Flexner report) 98% of the schools of nursing in the United States were "under the absolute control, both physical and financial, of the hospitals with which they are associated"(1, p. 971). This state of affairs created some peculiar dilemmas for nursing education. Hospitals were in the business of caring for the sick. Schools were supposed to educate their students. Nursing students, however, comprised the bulk of the nursing staffs at the hospitals where they were supposedly being educated. Indeed, the nursing student operated in a "Catch 22" situation.

> Doctors whose first thought and interest most naturally are centered upon the care and welfare of their patients become bitterly resentful when student nurses are taken from heavy wards to attend classes and condemn such practice in no uncertain terms. (What patients think about it has never been ascertained.) Under existing circumstances just how nursing education is other wise to be acquired, no one ever tells us. The only doctors who are at all patient with us are the ones who do the lecturing. It must be said, however, that the very doctors who do the most fussing about students being taken off the wards to attend classes are the first ones to protest when a graduate nurse is sent them who appears ignorant or shows a lack of adequate technical knowledge in connection with her nursing tasks(1, p. 972).

Even though nurses presented a strong case for fiscal, administrative, and educational autonomy of nursing schools at the AHA meeting, the two physicians who presented their views were less enthusiastic. Dr. Doane, the director of a municipal hospital, reviewed the pros and cons of autonomy for nursing schools and seemed supportive but ended his remarks with the sentence, "Finally it is a weighty obligation indeed to admit young women to training schools for education but it is to me a far more serious thing to admit a sick man to a hospital unless he can be properly treated"(14).

KOAN

Discuss the remark made by Dr. Doane. Does it support autonomy for the nursing school? Does it hint at an anti-intellectualist view of nursing education?

Dr. Howland, the medical director of a hospital, who also spoke on the question of autonomy for nursing schools, stressed the economic problems that a hospital would encounter if "the training school were strictly on an educational basis"(15). He predicted the inevitable growth of central schools of nursing connected with colleges and universities that would supply nurses to the smaller hospitals. This was an idea that had been discussed as an option by nursing leaders for some time.

At the same meeting Annie Goodrich stressed the need in nursing education for a foundation in the sciences, which, she felt, was best obtained through a college or university. She believed that one hospital or institution could not provide the broad range of experience needed for the care of the sick and for primary prevention. Goodrich recommended two types of schools from which nursing education could best be obtained. ". . . the university school of nursing and the so-called central schools of nursing. Through either one, the small hospitals desiring a student body can be effectively served. Such institutions can either make the preliminary or preclinic term a prerequisite for enrollment, or can enroll their students and then, through scholarship or other means provide for the preliminary course"(16).

Goodrich emphasized that the success of such an educational system for nursing would depend on hospitals budgeting for paid graduates to staff their nursing services and students paying for their own educations while being reimbursed for their services. A series of studies and reports (see Table 5-2) from 1923 to the present reinforced the concept that nursing education belongs in institutions of higher learning.

By 1938 hospitals still controlled the majority of nursing schools, but collegiate programs for nurses had grown steadily. Petry reported that in 1938 there were 70 basic nursing curricula in 66 institutions of higher learning(17). World War II brought an increase in the number of collegiate schools of nursing. Nursing departments in colleges and universities were viewed as an economic asset in light of decreased enrollments caused by the war.

In 1952 the first associate degree programs opened in junior colleges, and they have grown more rapidly than any other type of

(Continued on page 160)

KOAN

One principle of change from a system's standpoint is that every change has its price. Before you proceed to the next section, list what you believe to be some of the benefits and deficits of nursing's move into academia.

Benefits	*Deficits*

Table 5–2. Summary of Recommendations From Selected Studies and Reports on Nursing Education and Health Manpower

Study	Recommendations
"The Goldmark Report" Josephine Goldmark *In Winslow,* CEA (ed.), *Nursing and Nursing Education in the U.S.* New York, The Macmillan Co., 1923.	Educational standards as accepted by the professions (and legislatively mandated by the more progressive states) must be maintained in the interest of public safety.
Nursing for the Future Esther Lucille Brown New York, Russell Sage Foundation, 1948.	Priorities should be placed on first establishing sound basic educational programs within institutions of higher learning before directing efforts to more advanced programs for graduate nurses. Competing diploma courses should be completely eliminated. *All resources and efforts should be directed toward building basic schools of nursing in universities and colleges, comparable in number, organization, and financial structure, with adequate facilities and distribution to serve the needs of the entire country.*
Education for Nursing Leadership Eleanor C. Lambertsen Philadelphia, J.B. Lippincott Co., 1958.	Professional nursing education should be a liberal education that is multidisciplinary stressing continuous learning and growth with the emphasis on problem solving—the process rather than the accumulation of facts—recognizing that the product of such a program is a beginning practitioner prepared to work toward an ideal and not just the current state of practice.

157

Table 5-2. (Continued)

Study	Recommendations
The Education of Nursing Technicians Mildred L. Montag New York: G.P. Putnam's Sons, 1951.	Differentiation in function of nursing practice would imply the need for differences in educational preparation, which would not support the ladder concept of advancing levels of education from the same foundation with similar objectives or goals. Students' learning experience should be based strictly upon educational principles and clearly separated from ward service and the theoretical work and learning laboratories. Teaching methods should be refined to accommodate larger numbers of students with limited numbers of qualified instructors in concentrated, shorter periods of time.
Educational Revolution in Nursing Martha E. Rogers New York, The Macmillan Co., 1961.	Curricula must be designed to support the primary purpose of professional education—to provide students with the principles and theories prerequisite to their practice. Educational leaders must spearhead a body of literature that will identify the theoretical concepts and provide the tests and scholarly research for such teaching.
Report of the National Advisory Commission on Health Manpower Washington, D.C., U.S Government Printing Office 1967-V. (Cit. No. 135442), 1967.	A national uniform licensing code should be developed for each category of health manpower requiring licensure to practice that would allow for greater mobility and standardization of practice.

Nurses should try to insure that the number of nurses admitted to the profession bears a close relationship to the employment demand for their services to "free its members from undue economic pressure."

Nurses, Patients and Pocketbooks
May Ayres Burgess
New York, '26 Committee on the Grading of Nursing Schools, 1928.

AMA accreditation standards for schools of medical technology should be amended to require college or university affiliation and large enough laboratories with qualified staff to provide adequate learning experience. Preclinical education should be strengthened, with increased emphasis on bacteriology, biochemistry, physics, and mathematics and with additional instruction in all aspects of quality control, instrumentation, and practical application of laboratory test results. There should be a certification examination that would evaluate the technician's knowledge, judgment, and proficiency in these areas, including further studies and site visits to determine if their education and practical performance meet the established criteria.

"National Correlations in Medical Technology Education"
In *Essentials*. AMA Dept. of Allied Medical Professions, 1969.

nursing program. Today the majority of nursing education programs are conducted in institutions of higher learning; community colleges, liberal arts colleges, and universities. There remain less than 300 accredited nursing programs under hospital control, and the growth of nursing programs for advanced degrees continues in academic settings. How has the move into academia served nursing and nursing education?

THE LEARNING ENVIRONMENT: FROM HOSPITAL TO ACADEMIA

Individuals and groups from both inside and outside the nursing profession continue to this day to question nursing education's move into academic settings. In fact, a recent nursing survey of more than 10,000 nurses revealed that 59.3% of the respondents believe that professional nurses should be educated in the hospital school(18). The NLN, the accrediting body for nursing education programs, recently reaffirmed its support of the four types of preservice programs—baccalaureate, associate degree, diploma, and practical nurse programs(19). In addition, the New York Academy of Medicine's Committee on Medical Education advocated in June 1977 a return to hospital school education where "a proper balance must be struck in nursing education between the patient's needs and the nurse's aspirations"(20). This committee also concluded that lengthy and expensive nursing education programs could discourage highly motivated applicants, especially those from "working class homes who are not paid to attend by welfare departments"(20, p. 500). This logic seems faulty in light of the fact that highly motivated people are usually not easily discouraged. Also, the committee of physicians seems not to have considered the length and expense of a medical education in comparison. This prestigious committee of physicians was also most concerned with the shift of nursing away from disease-oriented care and the hospital environment, which is certainly a physician-dominated one. "Neglect of direct care of patients," said the New York committee, "in favor of emphasis on academic education has weakened and may destroy hard-earned gains by generations of dedicated, idealistic people who became nurses primarily to serve, not to gain status"(20, p. 505).

KOAN

Can the caring role of nursing coexist with the seeking of professional status?

In the face of so much opposition, it is a testament to the tenacity of the nursing education system that it has flourished in academic settings at all.

What did the nursing education leaders of the early 1900s hope to accomplish in a collegiate setting that could not be accomplished in a hospital setting? Was their aim to produce a more polished product, a leader or a "super nurse," while the hospital school trained ordinary practitioners to do the work of nursing? Stewart, who raised this question in 1940, asserted that one aim of the collegiate school of nursing was to "prepare better *practitioners* on all levels for the many different fields of nursing service," but a more important goal was to "produce a richer, freer, and more rounded and integrated personality. We do not expect these (collegiate) nurses will show greater technical skill than the nurses who receive the older type of training, but we believe that they should be better able to think out their problems to meet varied and unpredictable demands of society in the future, and to become self-reliant, self-directing, growing professional women (and men)"(21).

Stewart advocated a system of nursing education that placed the development of the student as a thinking, multifaceted individual *before* the needs of the patient and the hospital environment, at least during the learning years. A nurse who had a liberal arts education, it was hoped, would ultimately raise the standards of practice and quality of care. These certainly were medicine's aims in revamping its educational system to require a baccalaureate degree even before entry into medical school. With a 700-year tradition of dedication to service, and with many collegiate nursing faculties imbued with the old traditions, has nursing successfully integrated practical education with liberal arts education? On the one hand, collegiate nursing education may be producing educated practitioners who do not fit into the traditional hierarchies of some practice settings as in the cases cited in

Chapter 4. On the other hand, collegiate programs may be producing nurses who do not *think* very well because of the crisis in the quality of education in American colleges and universities and who do not practice very well because of a dearth of clinical experience in the preservice program and a lack of practicing role models as faculty(22). The Rush-Presbyterian University School of Nursing in Chicago uses a matrix system to avoid the latter problem. The faculty is made up of expert clinicians with clinical case loads who integrate teaching with practice. Students learn to nurse by working with and observing these faculty clinicians. The Rush system strives for a balance between theory and practice.

Stewart was concerned with achieving balance in nursing education between a liberal education and a practical education(21, p. 1035). Can collegiate nursing education harmonize the following factors?

· individual development and concern for the general well-being of the student
· interest and effort
· freedom and duty
· theory and practice
· independent thinking and respect for authority
· liberal education and technical training
· preparation of the nurse and preparation of the individual
· democracy, discipline and efficiency

KOAN

How far has collegiate education progressed in harmonizing the above factors? Where is there balance? Where is there imbalance? Use your own collegiate programs or those you know as a model for discussing these questions. (*Collegiate* refers to associate degree, baccalaureate, and higher degree programs.)

Can the academic setting in its present state of evolution within a changing society still hope to blend these elements in nursing education? Has nursing been unrealistic in its hopes that a change of educational setting from hospital to academia would ensure the maximizing of nursing's potential?

The structure of American universities and colleges closely resembles that of the hospital. The models depicted in Fig. 5-3 of the organizational hierarchy of a university and a hospital are comparable.

The hierarchical structure of the American university or college is certainly not comparable to the participatory democracies of Oxford, Cambridge, and other European universities, where students often dominate university policy. In today's college or university, administrators and regents can overrule faculty councils and departments, since it is in the administration that ultimate power lies. "Students and staff have little formal power in the organization"(23). If both hospital and university are hierarchical systems, what, then, is the advantage of moving nursing education into academia?

The most obvious advantage in nursing's move to academia is the faculty's control over curriculum development and teaching within the framework of the university philosophy, which is in most cases liberal. The collegiate faculty concentrates on preparing a health professional to practice in the future in a constantly changing health care delivery system. The hospital school faculty may have the same lofty aims, but there is always at least subtle pressure to produce a nurse who will also be a model employee. Despite the quality of the faculty and the excellence of curricula, there is bound to be some conflict of interest when an employing institution, the hospital, attempts to educate members of a profession. This conflict of interest often restricts the faculty's

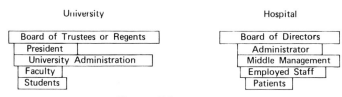

Figure 5-3.

freedom to experiment with new nursing roles and functions, to depart from the medical model (see Chap. 6), and to discuss controversial nursing issues that might make the nursing student a "troublesome" future employee.

A hospital school of nursing faculty had recently voted to include in the maternal/child-health course several lectures and demonstrations on the importance of continuous gynecological self-assessment for women of all ages. The lecturer, a nurse clinician from an inner-city neighborhood health center, delivered the lectures and demonstrations and was paid with visiting lecturer funds from the nursing school budget. Two weeks after the clinician's presentation the chief physician of the obstetrical department interrupted a faculty meeting, accused the faculty of condoning the illegal practice of medicine by "this nurse clinician"; and threatened the director of the school with termination of employment. The administrator of the hospital reassured the director of the school that she would not be fired since the physician had no authority to terminate her employment. The hospital administrator did, however, encourage the director to use "more discretion" in inviting "outsiders" to teach in the school in the future.

A collegiate nursing program contracted with a nearby hospital nursing department to provide the clinical laboratory for an obstetrical experience that was part of a family health nursing course. There were two male nursing students in the first group of seven students to use the obstetrical unit during the fall semester. Several members of the medical staff questioned the propriety of having male nurses in the delivery room. One physician banned male nursing students from "his" delivery room. After unsuccessful negotiations with the physician, the faculty member reported the incident to the curriculum coordinator who had negotiated the contract with the hospital nursing department. Because the college nursing department had been granted federal funds, a clause in every contract with clinical facilities stated that both the college and the hospital agreed to provide equal educational opportunities to all

students. The hospital honored their commitment when informed of the situation.

A hospital school faculty revised the curriculum so that an
independent study issues seminar was part of the senior
program. Each student chose an issue to explore, wrote his
or her own objectives, and negotiated a learning contract
with the faculty member. One student chose to explore the
issue of collective bargaining. As part of her project she
arranged to interview the hospital personnel director and a
licensed practical nurse who was believed to be a union
organizer. There was no union in the hospital at the time.
Two weeks after the student completed the project, the personnel director visited the director of the school and asked
why the faculty was teaching the nursing students to
unionize. He cautioned the director to "tighten the reigns"
on the faculty's freedom. "Remember," he said, "this is a
hospital, not the Berkeley campus!"

KOAN

After discussing the above cases, list other subjects that might be taboo in a hospital school setting. List curricula issues that might be taboo in a
collegiate setting, including a community college
setting. Which list is longer? Why?

Moving nursing education into academia is certainly no guarantee of escape from the domination of medicine. Collegiate schools
of nursing that are part of schools of health sciences might experience pressures similar to hospital school faculties, particularly if the health science school is medically dominated. In matters of curriculum planning and decision-making, however, there
is considerably more freedom for nursing faculty in academic
rather than in service settings.

The importance of freedom for a nursing faculty was reported
in a study by Marriner and Craigie(24). In an investigation of job
satisfaction and mobility of nurse educators from 36 accredited

baccalaureate and higher degree programs they found that faculty "ranked intrinsic factors—such as responsibility, achievement, academic freedom, and autonomy" as highly important in a teaching position(24, p. 353). They also found a high correlation between an open organizational climate and job satisfaction and between a closed organizational climate and job dissatisfaction.

Increased freedom and autonomy for nurse educators is, of course, no guarantee of teaching or program excellence. Freedom must always be balanced with accountability, particularly in the marketplace of the university where the student is the consumer. This accountability dictates that nursing faculty continually rethink and reaffirm the central purpose of nursing and its commitment to society. This process is more easily accomplished in an academic setting than in a hospital where commitments are more localized and less future oriented. Academia, however, is by no means a utopian setting. In fact, a university or college, with its diverse subsystems (departments), can lose sight of its purpose. "Sociologists point out that over the years most institutions develop a kind of inner momentum having little to do with their ostensible purpose ... much of what goes on in hospitals, for instance, has almost nothing to do with the fact that they contain ... patients"(*The Village Voice*, August 23, 1976, p. 56).

The unique problems of contemporary colleges and universities can work against the aims of nursing education as was the case with hospitals in the first half of this century. Boulding, a university educator, noted economist, and social ecologist, believes that "one of the major problems of the university is the weakness of its ostensibly primary function—teaching. It is universally admitted that university teaching is pedestrian and ill rewarded . . ."(23, p. 300). Because the results of teaching are so difficult to evaluate and so invisible in the college system, research and publication are used as criteria for promotion or salary increases. This system, Boulding asserts, does not guarantee quality teaching. "Even attempts at student evaluation (of faculty) are by no means conclusive, as a student often discovers that he had a good teacher only when he has graduated and is no longer accessible to questionnaires"(23, p. 301).

Collegiality among university faculty, particularly within the departmental system, can also work against excellence in teaching. The great economist, Adam Smith, noted at Oxford that collegiality* and egalitarianism within universities can easily lead faculty members into excusing each other's inactivity and forgoing progress for peace and security. "This is the great principle of the convoy going at the pace of the slowest ship. Individualism in the market produces inequality and progress: collegiality produces equality and stagnation"(23, p. 300).

KOAN

As a student, are you or were you a higher achiever, an individualist among your student peers? Do you or did you forego distinguished achievement for the sake of collegiality?

Dwindling funds, declining enrollments, and negative social forces are influencing every aspect of higher education(25). The disenchantment with a liberal arts education that does not prepare students for jobs may serve to strengthen the position of nursing departments within institutions of higher education. Strong nursing departments that strike a balance among teaching, research, and service can develop innovative nursing curricula that will blend liberal education with human service and will be blueprints for the actions of future nurses.

LEARNING AND RELEVANCE: THE CURRICULUM

In a 1977 issue of the *Journal of Medical Education,* a physician-author proposed a model for teaching comprehensive health care. This model is very similar to what Nightingale proposed in 1859. The physician states, "It is the responsibility of medical educators to acquaint students with the advantages of assessing the patient's total needs and of utilizing a broad range of services to assist the patient in achieving the fullest health potential"(26).

*The pretense that one's native abilities and level of expertise are the same.

His model for teaching comprehensive health care uses a three-dimensional approach with the individual, the family, and the community as the data bases; physical, psychological, and sociological assessment parameters; and curative, preventive, and health-promoting plans of action.

KOAN

Compare the above model for teaching health care to medical students with the way nursing leaders have defined the purpose of nursing for the past 100 years. (See Table 1-1.) What conclusions might you draw from such a comparison?

In 1912 the Flexner report urged the adoption of the strict scientific-research orientation as a curriculum model for medical schools. "Science aims toward human mastery of world and self through expanding of powers of prediction and control ... It breaks problems into components, figures out their functional relations, places them under schemes of prediction and control and thus reduces them to human power"(27). To be sure, science has and will continue to make strides. However, the scientific models that attempt to reduce living organisms to their individual parts and then to treat each part separately, losing sight of the whole, are reaching the limits of their usefulness.

More than 50 years after embracing the pure science-oriented medical model, medicine is beginning to see the virtue in viewing a person as a unified entity. In 1976, for example, Christie reported that the trend in undergraduate curricula in medical education was toward integrated teaching in which the medical curriculum was taught by interdepartmental teams. "Teaching is based on organs or systems, each department giving its contribution, so that the student is presented with a complete picture of the system usually including its application"(28). This means that at least by 1976 physician-professors from the renology department were talking about the kidney's relationship to the heart with physician-professors from the cardiology department.

The American medical school worked on integrating the body in the curricula of the 70s, while the curricula in nursing schools continued to view the person as a unified whole—mind, body, and spirit—in dynamic interaction with health instead of illness as the focus.

But has the evolution of nursing curricula up to the present provided the nursing student with a "relevant" education in light of the demands of the present health care system? This question can be answered from two perspectives. From the perspective of the demands of the health care system, current nursing curricula, with their health-oriented, total person-family focus, may not seem relevant. Such a curriculum does not produce a nurse who can immediately adapt to the work demands of the acute care setting. An extended period of orientation or internship is needed, sometimes at a cost of $1,000 to $3,000 per nurse(29). From the perspective of health care trends and projections (see Chap. 6), current integrated nursing curricula may be more relevant than any other professional health-related curricula. It depends on one's point of view. A nursing curriculum serves as a template, or pattern, from which a nurse expands the theory and practice base. No degree is ever the final step in education. In fact, the continuing education system in nursing is experiencing a period of great expansion.

KOAN

Is the nursing curriculum that serves as the basis of your undergraduate education relevant to what you believe to be nursing's central purpose?

CONTINUING EDUCATION: A KOAN

Continuing education for nurses (CEN) is not new. However, its importance to nursing practice is a current issue. Nurses have always shown an interest in continued learning for their own professional growth. The first formal continuing education program for the practicing nurse originated in 1894, although even before this the alumnae associations of nursing schools had provided social and educational opportunities for their graduates. Alumnae associations can, therefore, be credited with offering the first form of continuing education for nurses(29).

An article in the first issue of the *American Journal of Nursing* in November, 1900, told of a group of nurses who had formed a literary club that "met once a fortnight and during the season many good papers were prepared and read by members, some of the subjects being 'Pneumonia,' 'Complications of Pneumonia,' 'Diptheria,' 'Croup,' and 'Ethics for Nurses.' " This was a voluntary group of professional nurses committed to the concept of lifelong learning(30).

Today, continuing education for nurses is mandatory in many states (see Table 5-3) in order to assure that practicing nurses are up-to-date in their knowledge and competencies. This has created a dilemma for the nursing profession. Although all nurses recognize the need for continued learning "to augment knowledge and skills necessary to enhance nursing practice, education, administration and research to improve health care to the public,"(30) when continuing education becomes linked to relicensure, a completely different issue is raised, the issue of competency to practice.

The U.S. Department of Health, Education, and Welfare has defined licensure as "the process by which an agency of government grants permission to an individual to engage in a given occupation upon finding that the applicant has attained the minimal degree of competency necessary to ensure that the public health, safety, and welfare will be reasonably protected"(31). The public, providers of health care, and the federal government have been exhorting each of the health professions to develop methods of demonstrating their members' continued competence to practice. In response, state legislators in many states have mandated continuing education as a precondition for renewal of licensure to practice. "Continuing education has been increasingly recognized as an essential way for nurses to expand their theoretical knowledge and enhance clinical performance"(32).

How can attendance at a certain number of continuing education programs of one's choice attest to continued competency to practice? How does continuing education protect the public from unsafe practitioners?

Table 5-3. Status of Mandatory CEN for Relicensure[a]

States That Have Laws Requiring Continuing Education for All Nurses

State	Date of Implementation	Required Number of Contact Hours	Subsequent Changes in Requirements
California	July 1, 1978	30 hours every 2 years	—
Colorado	January 1, 1980	20 hours every 2 years	—
Florida	March 1, 1981	30 hours every 2 years	—
Iowa	January 1, 1980	Not yet determined	—
Kansas	July 1, 1978	5 hours in 1 year	15 hours every 2 years after June 30, 1980; then 30 hours every 2 years after June 30, 1982
Kentucky	April 30, 1982	5 hours in 1 year	10 hours in 1983 and 15 hours in 1984
Massachusetts	June 1, 1982	5 hours every year in 1982–1983	10 hours yearly in 1984 and 1985; 15 hours yearly after 1985
Minnesota	August 1, 1980	15 hours every 2 years	30 hours every 2 years after August 1, 1980
Nebraska	January 1, 1981	Not yet determined	—
New Mexico	January 1, 1981	30 hours every 2 years	—

States in Which the Boards of Nursing Have Rules and Regulations That Permit Them to Require Continuing Education
Michigan, North Dakota, South Dakota

States That May Require a Certain Category of Nurses to Engage in Continuing Education Activity
Alaska, Delaware, Louisiana, New Hampshire, Oregon, Utah

[a] For specific requirements, refer to ANA's *Mandatory Continuing Education: The Legislative State of the Art. A Resource Paper.* Kansas City, Missouri, American Nurses Association, April, 1979.

171

Cooper has suggested that the issue of relicensure be separated from continuing education because "if you believe there is a rationale for a licensing examination in the first place, it may make sense to require another examination at 5-year intervals . . ."(33). Nursing leaders in states that have not yet established mandatory continuing education are asking if this is the way to ensure competency. Many proponents of mandatory status for CEN believe that it will stimulate action toward the establishment and acceptance of uniform CEN standards and prompt the development of more educationally sound CEN programs.

KOAN

Is nursing's attempt to perfect a system of continuing education for professional nurses an overcompensation for its lack of success in standardizing the preservice nursing education system?

Mandatory continuing education is that education necessary to meet legal requirements. Since the United States Constitution grants each state the right to determine licensing standards, it is the legislature in each state that will determine whether and how much continuing education will be required for relicensure. Consequently, requirements for relicensure will vary from state to state, adding to the confusion and making reciprocity very difficult for nurses who relocate (see Table 5-3). It is questionable whether the fulfillment of continuing education requirements should be equated with competency and automatically qualify the applicant for relicensure.

Evaluation, according to Knowles, is a static concept(34). Instead of thinking in terms of assessing the results of learning, he advocates thinking more in terms of rediagnosing learning needs. At the end of a learning experience, he asks adult students to reexamine their models of required competencies and reassess their levels of development in particular areas. "Two things happen: they [the adult learners] discover that they have raised their levels of aspiration regarding the required competencies and that new gaps have appeared between where they are now and where they want to be in their development. Rediagnosing thus builds in the notion of continued learning, which I think the static concept of evaluation largely destroys"(34, p. 35).

When continuing education for relicensure first became an issue in 1971, the ANA established a task force to study the concepts of voluntary continuing education as a professional responsibility and mandatory continuing education as a requirement for renewal of licensure. A council of continuing education was established at the same time to determine the ANA's role in continuing education and to develop standards and program guidelines for continuing education in nursing. The *Standards for Continuing Education in Nursing,* published in 1974, were applicable to both mandatory and voluntary systems. The ANA also assumed responsibility for the regulation and accreditation of these programs, even though many of them were being provided by nonacademic institutions that had no provisions for evaluating educational quality. The ANA's accreditation mechanism for continuing education covers local, state, regional, and national programs.

The NLN, since its inception, has also been committed to continuing education in nursing through its council programs and workshops. The NLN "assumes full responsibility for the establishment of criteria and evaluation of continuing education offerings located in those nursing education and service programs that the NLN accredits. Educational offerings within a school of nursing or health agency are interrelated; since the quality of one program of a school or agency necessarily affects the quality of other programs, it is important that the NLN Councils retain responsibility for the accreditation of educational activities"(35).

Thus, two accrediting bodies, the ANA and the NLN, assume the responsibility for establishing criteria for and evaluation of continuing education programs within a school of nursing. In addition, each state board of nursing is free to establish its own criteria where CEN is mandatory. The future promises no lack of criteria for continuing education.

Continuing education for nursing is caught in a maze of accreditation procedures. The awarding of credentials to health personnel, which includes accreditation of programs, certification for special competencies, licensure, and an academic degree, is an attempt to foster acceptable performance in people and education and service programs. Many sociopolitical factors influence practices. For example, ". . . allegations of anticompetitive practices have recently been lodged against the health field, raising issues and concerns that are usually associated with big business. This has come about because antitrust enforcers of the Federal Trade Commission view health care as big business and question its profits. . . . The demand for greater public representation in accreditation of professional schools and in occupational licensing will affect nurses as well as other professionals"(36).

In 1975 the ANA appointed an independent study committee to investigate the feasibility of devising accreditation mechanisms for basic and graduate nursing programs in view of the changing social climate. The first report of this two-year study, called "The Study of Credentialing in Nursing: A New Approach," is aimed at the utterly confusing situation in nursing's many accrediting bodies and recommends that ". . . a national nursing credentialing center be established as the means of achieving a unified, coordinated, comprehensive credentialing system for nursing" for the purpose of studying, developing, coordinating, and providing services for and conducting the awarding of credentials in nursing(37). When continuing education is viewed apart from its role as a prerequisite for relicensure, it loses its monstrous image and regains its status as a legitimate vehicle for adult learning.

There are basic differences between adult learning principles called andragogy and those most commonly used in nursing education programs, which are more closely allied to pedagogy—the teaching of children. Essentially these are the differences:

1. Adults want to be self-directed and assume responsibility for their own learning, whereas pedagogical learning is teacher directed. Therefore, adults need to participate in the planning and decision-making that is often assumed by the teacher.
2. Adult learning is essentially task- or problem-centered, related to current needs, and not curriculum- or subject-centered, with an orientation to the future.
3. Adults are motivated by the demands of a task or feelings of inadequacy in coping, indicating a need for further preparation or learning. Knowles calls this "reexamining their models of required competencies and reassessing their levels of development"(34). Diagnoses of learner needs are more often

achieved by mutual assessment rather than primarily by the teacher. The adult is assumed to be motivated by internal incentives and curiosity rather than by external rewards or punishment. "He'll be ready to inquire into these areas of content as he confronts problems to which they are relevant"(34, p. 39).

4. Adults bring a reservoir of experience that accumulates and becomes an increasing resource for learning.

When these principles of adult education are ignored in professional continuing education programs, it is little wonder that nurses experience growing dissatisfaction. Professional nurses do not question the need for continuing education in nursing. Lifelong learning is an accepted criteria for any profession.

General guidelines, standards, and criteria for evaluating CEN have been established by the ANA on a national level to help interstate recognition of acceptable continuing education activities. These guidelines may be interpreted differently by the separate state nursing associations when they apply these criteria to programs seeking their approval. Some state councils of continuing education are overzealous in their attempt to apply the standards and have become unnecessarily restrictive. How can nursing demand evidence of acquired learning in CEN when nursing has not yet demonstrated acquired competencies in formal nursing education? Nursing has yet to develop valid tools for measuring the effectiveness of continuing education. Until such tools have been developed, it is unreasonable to demand evidence for such effectiveness from CEN sponsors.

KOAN

Several nurses attend a continuing education program that has been approved by the state nurses' association. At the end of the program the nurses are given a test related to the content of the program to measure the learning they have accomplished that day. Discuss the pros and cons of this method of evaluation.

It has not yet been proved that continuing education improves patient care even though it is a recognized means by which nurses expand their theoretical knowledge and enhance clinical practice. It cannot yet be claimed that CEN assures competency to practice at a time when all methodologies for assessing competence need to undergo further research and development. The "Study on Credentialing in Nursing" states, "Competence, like quality, is a dynamic concept that changes over time; it is based on expanding knowledge, changing technology, reordering of priorities, and redefinition of values. An academic degree or certificate of completion of a program has a static, rather than a dynamic quality, and although these have high value for assessing entry competence they lose value in assessing continued competence"(37, p. 61). Much more research is needed on the relationship of CEN to improved client/patient care.

Self-directed CEN is an option for many nurses in geographically isolated areas where the type of program desired is not readily available or for those who are homebound and unable to attend formal CEN programs. Opportunities for self-directed learning activities are now almost limitless with telephone-dial access systems, television, computer-assisted instruction, audio and video cassette lectures and courses, programmed instruction packages, and the increasing number of current periodicals in the health care field.

The essence of adult education is self-directed learning. For many this is the preferred, the most effective, method for learning. A self-directed learning activity may be designed by the learner or by others (as in formats listed above). To receive credit or recognition for a self-directed learning activity, documentation is required from the learner. The ANA has developed guidelines and criteria for approving self-designed, self-directed learning that should help the interstate transferability of continuing education records(38).

With guidelines for the self-design process (planning, implementation, evaluation, and documentation), more nurses may be willing to consider self-directed learning as a legitimate form of continuing education. This is the one method that takes into account individual learning styles and allows students to proceed at their own pace according to their individual learning needs. Some states already have well-defined guidelines for approval of self-directed learning activities. Nurses seeking recognition for an independent learning project where CEN is mandatory are advised to consult their state nurses' association or licensing body.

Continuing education in nursing is an issue of major concern and complexity, since it represents a microcosm of all other issues in nursing. CEN can be viewed as a series of KOANS for the reader to discuss and debate and to use as the impetus to revise the system.

KOAN

What is continuing education in nursing? Does your view coincide with what is depicted on Table 5-4?

Can CEN be adequately defined without a clear delineation of the central purpose of nursing?

How can the nursing profession assume the responsibility for maintaining standards of practice when control of licensure is fragmented and is defined by each state separately?

How can nursing strike a balance between uniformity and rigidity in its efforts to design systems that recognize and give credit for continuing education?

Who should determine the needs for specific continuing educational programs? *(1)* The nurse participant who requests such programs? *(2)* The provider of health services (other than nurses, e.g., health administrators) who identify the need for special services or expanding the nurses' role? or, *(3)* The consumer of health care who desires alternate approaches to care giving practices?

Should a formal collective bargaining agent like the ANA also be an accrediting body of continuing education programs? Is there a conflict of interest?

(Continued on page 180)

Table 5–4. What Is Continuing Education in Nursing?

A Variety of Learning Experiences (Beyond Basic Preparation for Nursing)	→	Offered by Various Institutions and Agencies or	→	For Numerous Reasons

Self-Directed Learning Activities

Program Content	→	Sponsoring Agencies	→	Philosophies
New products		Commercial programmers (RoCom—Conedics) and proprietary firms (drug and supply firms)		Commercial services—updating practice
New techniques				
New or updated skills				
New knowledge		Single-purpose health agencies or special interest groups		Improvement in standards of practice and quality of care
New areas of practice				
Improved patient teaching-learning		Health service agencies		Preparation for changing roles and functions
New techniques in leadership-management		Hospitals—acute care institutes		
New teaching tools and techniques		Long-term—extended care—rehab centers		Expansion of professional education—for certification of specialty practice
New theories—curricula		Community health care agencies		
Application of research findings in education in nursing practice		Hospital schools of nursing		Promotion of research in nursing theory and practice
		Health foundations		

Biomedical/ethical issues
Sociopolitical issues of health care
Health legislation
Politics of change
Patient advocacy

Professional organizations
National and state nursing groups
Specialty groups in nursing
Organizations for other health disciplines

Governmental agencies
Department of Health
Department of Higher Education
Department of Law—Public Safety

Institutions of higher learning
Colleges
Universities

Improvement in health care delivery system
Improvement in interdisciplinary/interdepartmental/consumer-public

179

> Should continuing education for professional
> growth and development be separate and distin-
> guishable from that which focuses solely on those
> competencies considered necessary for a safe
> level of practice?
>
> As the pressure for continuing education in nurs-
> ing increases, so will the cost. Who should pay?
> How much would you be willing to spend a year
> on your own continuing education?

A recent nursing survey indicated that hospitals are caught between nurses' increasing demands for continuing education and
the public outcry against rising costs. The results indicated that
hospitals may be showing a trend toward tightening their policies
rather than responding to the demand for more CEN. Thirty-
seven percent of the respondents said that they received no pay or
reimbursement for CEN courses(39).

The issues surrounding CEN will probably become even more
obscure as "a large number of organizations, groups, and private
companies with widely varying qualifications have rushed in as
providers of CEN . . . to meet the demand for programs and in
some cases to turn a tidy profit"(40). Each nurse will have to
come to terms with the commitment of time and money that may
be required to maintain a desired level of practice. This will demand attention to and close scrutiny of the burgeoning market in
continuing education offerings. Each nurse must select carefully
what is best suited to individual and professional needs to get the
most out of the educational dollar, since "an inexpensive program
may not be a bargain and a high price is not a guarantee of
quality"(40, p. 38).

The primary goal of any learning system is to develop people to
the point where they are intrinsically motivated to seek new
knowledge. The nursing education system at its best will equip its
learners to meet and to create new challenges and to develop into
versatile professionals who can respond to creative innovations in
the health care system.

REFERENCES

1. Greener EA, Goodrich AW, Doane JC, et al: Shall the school of nursing have autonomy? *Am J Nurs* 28:986, 1928.

2. Meyer JW, Rowan B: Institutionalized organizations: formal structure as myth and ceremony. *American Journal of Sociology* 83:340–363, 1977.

3. Parsons T, Platt G: *The American University.* Cambridge, Mass., Harvard University Press, 1975, p 226.

4. Stewart I: *The Education of Nurses.* New York, Macmillan Inc, 1944, pp 23–24.

5. Waite FC: *The First Medical College in Vermont: Castleton 1818–1862.* Montpelier, Vermont, 1949, pp 57–58.

6. Hudson RP: Abraham Flexner in perspective: American medical education 1865–1910. *Bull Hist Med* pp 545–561, 1972.

7. Fishbein M: *A History of the American Medical Association: 1847–1947.* Philadelphia, WB Saunders Company, 1947, p 243.

8. Stevens P: *American Medicine and the Public Interest.* New Haven, Yale University Press, 1971, p 55.

9. Nutting A, Dock L: *A History of Nursing,* New York, GP Putnam's Sons, 1912, vol II, p 182.

10. Nightingale F: Suggestions for the improvement of the nursing service of hospitals and on the method of training nurses for the sick poor, in Nutting A, Dock L, *A History of Nursing,* New York, GP Putnam's Sons, 1912, vol II, p 182.

11. Marshall H: *Mary Adelaide Nutting: Pioneer of Modern Nursing.* Baltimore, The John's Hopkins University Press, 1972, p 87.

12. O'Hanlon G: The responsibility of the hospital to the school of nursing. *Am J Nurs* 28:784, 1928.

13. West RH: *History of Nursing in Pennsylvania.* Harrisburg, Pennsylvania, Pennsylvania Nurses Association, 1926, p 123.

14. Doane JC: Shall the school of nursing have autonomy? From the standpoint of the municipal hospital. *Am J Nurs* 28:986, 1928.

15. Howland JB: Shall the school of nursing have autonomy? From the standpoint of the medical director of the hospital. *Am J Nurs* 28:978, 1928.

16. Goodrich A: Shall the school of nursing have autonomy? *Am J Nurs* 28:978, 1928.

17. Petry L: Basic professional curricula in nursing leading to degrees. *Am J Nurs* 37:287, 1937.

18. Lee A: Seven out of ten nurses oppose the professional technical split. *RN* 42:83–93, 1979.

19. National League for Nursing: *Position Statement on Preparation for Beginning Practice in Nursing.* New York, National League for Nursing, February, 1979, Pub. No. 11-1772.

20. Committee on Medical Education of the New York Academy of Medicine: Statement on nursing education: Status or service oriented. *Bull NY Acad Med* 53:500, 1977.

21. Stewart I: The philosophy of the collegiate school of nursing. *Am J Nurs* 40:1034–35, 1940.

22. Graubard S (ed): American higher education: Toward an uncertain future. *Daedalus* 104, 1975.

23. Boulding K: Quality vs. equality, the dilemma of the university in American higher education: Toward an uncertain future. *Daedalus,* 104:299, 1975.

24. Marriner A, Craigie D: Job satisfaction and mobility of nursing educators. *Nurs Res* 26:349–360, 1977.

25. Graubard S (ed): American higher education: Toward an uncertain future. *Daedalus* 104, 1975.

26. Smilkstein G: A model for teaching comprehensive health care. *J Med Educ* 52:773–775, 1977.

27. Novak M: The liberation of imagination. *Man and Medicine* 1:97, 1976.

28. Christie RV: *Medical Education and the State.* NIH 76-943 US Department of Health, Education and Welfare, 1976.

29. Kramer M, Schmalenberg CE: Dreams and reality: Where do they meet? *J Nurs Adm* 6:35–43, May 1976.

29. Flanagan L: *One Strong Voice: The Story of the American Nurses Association.* Kansas City, American Nurses Association Publishing and Lowell Press, 1976, p 253.

30. Council on Continuing Education, Revised definition of continuing education for nurses. American Nurses Association, August, 1978.

31. Report on licensure and related health personnel credentialing. No. 72-11 US Department of Health, Education and Welfare, Office of Assistant Secretary for Health and Scientific Affairs, 1971, p 7.

32. Mandatory continuing education: The legislative state of the art, a Resource paper. Kansas City, American Nurses Association, April 1979, p 1.

33. Hochman G: Mandatory continuing education: How will it affect you? *Nursing '78* 8:113, 1978.

34. Knowles MS: Innovations in teaching styles and approaches based upon adult learning, *Journal of Education for Social Work,* 8:39, 1972.

35. Position statement on NLN's role in continuing education in nursing. National League for Nursing, November, 1975.

36. Federal trade commission seeks competition in health field. *Public Affairs Advisory,* National League for Nursing, March 1979.

37. *The study of credentialing in nursing: A new approach.* Kansas City, American Nurses Association, January 1979, vol 1, p 91.

38. *Self-directed Continuing Education in Nursing.* American Nurses Association, Kansas City, Missouri, 1978.

39. Donovan L: Who's going to pay for all that continuing education? *RN* 41:48–51, 1978.

40. Del Bueno D: How to get your money's worth out of continuing education. *RN* 41:37–42, April 1978.

CHAPTER SIX

Delphi for Nursing

> All the secrets of your foundation must come to light; when you are uprooted and broken in the sun your lie will be separable from your truth.
>
> *Nietzsche*
> Thus Spake Zarathustra

CHANGING PASTS—ALTERNATIVE FUTURES

It is natural for people to try to foretell the future. The ancient Greeks consulted the oracle at Delphi in an effort to predict and control future events. The oracle, however, did not predict with precision and clarity. The messages were cryptic, vague, and ambiguous. The oracle gave hints that the person could use in alternative ways. Today we have computers and sophisticated data-analysis methods. However, forecasting the future still cannot be done with precision, since the components of any system are changing as they interact with each other and with the environment. Even our knowledge and beliefs about the past are changing. In fact, nursing's past, which at one time many believed to be an objective reality, is now being viewed from several perspectives. For example, many accounts of nursing's history are now being viewed from a feminist perspective such as in Ashley's *Hospitals, Paternalism and the Role of the Nurse*(1) and Ehrenreich's and English's *Witches, Midwives and Nurses*(2). These accounts

185

of the past do indeed differ from many other interpretive accounts of the past. They are no less true, however, for in many ways the past is just as elusive as the future.

Interpretations of the nursing system's development within larger systems are important to consider before attempting to construct alternative futures. From a systems perspective, "past reckoning is inseparable from future reckoning, because we need to make very strong and effective judgments about the future in order to be able to use the past effectively . . . The reverse is also clear . . . effective reckoning of the past is essential because effective judgments about the future of the system must somehow draw on past experience"(3). Before reckoning with nursing's possible futures, a coherent view of the past is required.

Past Reckoning*

The High Middle Ages was one of the most crucial periods in the formation of our modern social and political institutions. The period from 1100 to 1400 A.D. saw the creation of the modern state and our system of representative government, the origins of our economic system, the rise of the university, and the beginnings of our professions—law, medicine, and nursing, to name but a few. All of these innovations today bear the marks of their medieval origin. They appeared in an age of collectivism rather than of individualism, of strongly delineated social and sexual hierarchies, and of intermingling of secular and religious concerns that were only just beginning to be separated. In no area is this influence more obvious than in the structure and perception of the nursing profession both from within the health care world and from society at large. Some of this inheritance is clearly positive, such as the sense of dedication most nurses feel in an age when to so many others their work is "just another job." And some of this inheritance is very harmful and contributes to the continuing inability of nurses, either as individuals or as a collectivity, to deal with themselves, with their health care colleagues, (chiefly doctors and administrators), and with lay society as members of a true profession—a self-regulating and self-perpetuating occupation whose members provide a skilled service to society. Before

*This section was contributed by P. Geary, Ph.D., Professor of History, Princeton University, and M. Geary, RN, M.S.N., formerly, Instructor of Nursing, Trenton State College.

nurses can act as change agents to deal effectively with these problems, they must understand the problems both in their present forms and from an historical perspective. An examination of the medieval origins of the nursing profession, intended neither to praise nor to condemn this past but simply to understand it, can thus be a step toward freeing nurses from those elements of their past that impede their future development.

Organized professional nursing has no direct history before the twelfth century for the simple reason that between the disappearance of urban life in the western world in late antiquity and the rebirth of towns, health care was provided in homes or at religious shrines. True, monasteries provided care to people from outside their communities, but this care was directed not to the sick but to travelers. The ill who traveled to religious shrines sought help not from the clergy but from the miraculous intervention of the saints.

This system of health care was perfectly suited to the needs of a rural, fragmented society possessing only the most basic knowledge of medicine and hygiene. No doubt families could provide as good or better care than anyone else, and maintenance of the sick at home reduced the chances of infection—a problem that made hospital care more lethal than home care until the nineteenth century. When towns began to reappear in the twelfth century, however, with their congestion, fragmented families, and large numbers of indigents, institutions designed to provide for the poor, both sick and well, likewise appeared. The nature of these foundations were, however, suited to an age whose social, medical, and mental systems differed radically from our own.

First, the primary purpose of these "hospitals" was not to provide for the sick but rather to save the souls of the charitable donors who founded them and of the men and women who staffed them. Since these institutions catered exclusively to the poor, the wealthy patrons had no personal need of the care these hospitals provided. Nor did the upper classes of the twelfth century have a "social conscience" that compelled them to improve the lot of those less fortunate than themselves. The poor and sick were that way because of divine will, and they were seen as useful because they provided an opportunity for good works. Likewise, the staff of those institutions, although lay women and men, looked upon their work first as a religious vocation leading them to salvation and second, frequently, as a means of sustaining themselves.

Thus the early documents and regulations of these hospitals are concerned almost exclusively with discussions of the lives and privileges of the staff and mention only in passing the patients, who would be viewed for more than two centuries as a means to an end and not an end in themselves.

Second, we have mentioned that these hospitals were staffed by lay men and women. Their status was something of an anomaly in a society in which the term *religious* applied only to people directly subject to the jurisdiction of the church, whose power in secular areas was enormous. Hospital staff members lived in common quarters for the most part (men and women separately), although the more wealthy among them could often live in their own houses. In an age when people who banded together without strict control by an established authority were mistrusted, this arrangement could not long endure and in fact disappeared in the following century.

If the actual religious status of the staff was unclear, the control of the institutions was clearly in the hands of the church. Charity of all sorts had traditionally been a function of the church, and, in northern Europe during the twelfth century, no other sort of public institution was sufficiently advanced to control such activities.

The actual care provided by these early hospitals was minimal and apparently directed without distinction to the poor, the sick, travelers, foundlings, women in labor, and so on. The physical plant consisted of a large, churchlike room in which patients, paupers, and pilgrims received a bed, food, religious services, and little else.

Increasing contact with the more civilized world of the eastern Mediterranean throughout the twelfth century brought about significant changes and improvements in European hospitals. A religious order of noblemen, the Knights of St. John Hospitalier (today the Knights of Malta), began specializing in the care of pilgrims, chiefly the sick, who arrived in Jerusalem. This order benefited from its contact with Eastern medicine and hospitals and developed the first systematic delivery of medical care by westerners. Pilgrims and crusaders were impressed with the order and upon their return to the West founded hospitals that they put in the hands of the Knights of St. John. Other religious orders, such as the Holy Ghost Order, founded about 1198, likewise began to appear across Europe and to provide hospital care of a more sophisticated nature than had hitherto been known.

The success of these hospitals founded by religious orders greatly affected the organization and function of privately founded hospitals. Their example and the enormously legalistic atmosphere of the thirteenth century brought about fundamental changes in the organization and lives of hospital personnel. First, the ambiguous nature of the staff's religious life was no longer tolerated. Members of the orders were religious. They had taken vows and lived by a common rule. Similarly, hospital staffs were required to abandon their lay status and adopt a rule, usually the Rule of St. Augustine, which provided the basis for the organization of many types of religious communities. Second, bishops and clerical administrators became increasingly concerned about sexual promiscuity, which they imagined was rampant among the male and female hospital workers. Hence rules provided elaborate procedures for preventing nurses, male and female, from associating with each other and for preventing female nurses from being alone with male patients. These sexual fears, directed primarily toward the women who were seen as the more active, aggressive seekers of sexual activity, along with a general increase in numbers of women seeking to join (or being forced into) religious orders, may account for the gradual feminization of nursing staffs. While in the twelfth century the sex ratio of hospital staffs had been roughly equal, the percentage of women increased steadily throughout the thirteenth century. Moreover, while the number of women increased, the remaining men took on duties that were increasingly administrative and clerical, while the women were restricted to staff positions.

The quality of thirteenth-century hospital care improved considerably over that of the century before. It consisted primarily of good food, personal hygiene, clean bed linens, and religious services. More medical treatments were provided, but these were done by physicians brought in from the outside by the hospital administration not by the nursing staff. Nursing training was haphazard and minimal, while by this time medicine was well established as a university-trained profession designed not for the salvation of the physician's soul but for the treatment of those who could afford it. In its organization, recruitment, training, and motivation, the medical profession could not have been more alien to the world of nursing.

Hospitals of the later Middle Ages faced the same problems encountered by hospitals today. The primary difficulty was financial. Throughout the thirteenth and fourteenth centuries, grants from founders were not often adequate to sustain hospitals. Inflation and increasing expenses for salaries of priests, physicians, servants, and bookkeepers, and most importantly, for food for patients and staff presented serious problems. Moreover, urban populations grew steadily throughout the first quarter of the fourteenth century, and the frequent epidemics, famines, and plagues of the rest of the century put enormous strains on hospital resources. Continuing income from donations, rents, inheritances from patients and staff, and even sale of clothing from patients who died in the hospitals was often inadequate to prevent bankruptcy.

As if things were not bad enough, this same period saw an increased tendency on the part of hospital personnel to attempt to divert as much of the hospital's resources as possible to their own support rather than to that of the sick. Since hospitals, like other religious foundations, were still viewed as being there primarily for the spiritual and material benefit of their founders and staff, it is not too surprising that numerous hospitals actually reduced the number of patients while continuing to live off the revenues of donations. By the fourteenth century, many hospitals had no more than one or two symbolic patients, and some had been transformed into cloistered convents of nuns providing care to no one but themselves.

As the fourteenth century progressed, however, the developing secular institutions of government were not happy with this state of affairs. Community administrations saw the care of the poor as a political necessity rather than as a means to the salvation of nurses' souls. Thus, when hospitals beset by financial difficulties turned to government for assistance, city fathers, themselves often businessmen experienced in efficient operation of large enterprises, took control of these institutions from the church and placed them under community control. This secularization of control was not, however, accompanied by laicization of staff. On the contrary, the town governments still considered the discipline of a religious order the best safeguard of women's honesty and morality. Thus the new secular administrations contented themselves with controlling financing, limiting the number of staff to the bare minimum, and the like, while insisting on the nurses' strict adherence to the religious rule.

By the end of the Middle Ages certain essential characteristics of Western nursing practice had been established. Nurses were religious women who had no control over their own lives, training, or the institutions they operated. Health care in general was controlled by a male medical profession from which nurses were excluded by their lack of a university education, and health care institutions were controlled by government administrators rather than by those most familiar with their operations. Finally, as a group, nurses were viewed with mistrust and erotic fascination by much of the public.

Nursing has changed enormously in the last six centuries, yet many of these characteristics, which evolved to suit the needs of a world so different from our own, continue to influence the profession. Nurses and laypersons alike still see nursing as a quasi-religious female vocation, and too often these traditions take precedence over nurses' own professional needs in areas such as education and financial rewards. Nursing still has no standard educational system according to which new professionals are trained, and, unlike the other professions such as law and medicine, nursing often allows outsiders such as academic administrators or physicians to have a preponderant voice in setting educational standards. Nursing practice, too, is still dominated by physicians, mostly male, and narrow-minded, cost-conscious hospital administrators who set nursing service priorities. And nurses still function largely within established organizations rather than by practicing independently or by founding their own health care organizations.

Were these difficulties clearly perceived by nurses themselves, the struggle to overcome them would not be so difficult. Unfortunately, too many nurses are themselves so imbued with traditions and assumptions from their medieval past that they fail to recognize how very arbitrary and limiting these traditions are and instead largely accept the handmaiden role they have inherited from the Middle Ages. Even most of the great reforms in the profession of the past 150 years here and abroad are still constrained by these ancient limits. But as nurses gain a better understanding of the archaic forces and attitudes that formed their profession, they can begin to recognize that what is now and has been in the past is neither always desirable nor necessary. Then they and their profession can grow from this historical past into a better and more useful future.

Future Reckoning

The future is a blending of past reckonings, current experiences, and hope. The sages claim that physical reality is an invention of mind. Can the future be invented in the minds of the present? The following is an alternative vision of the nursing and health care system for the year 2025. Such a projection, based on past trends and current technological advances is designed to transcend the weight of daily obstacles that often inhibit creative visions of the future.

KOAN

Read the following projection of the future. Revise it according to your own projections or beliefs about the future. Become aware of how much past experience and habit is influencing your projections.

In the year 2025, hospitals as they are structured today will no longer exist. There will be no need for them. Emergency medical service will be available via mobile treatment centers. Technology with its advanced biomedicine and therapeutics will make surgery very rapid; tissue adhesives will have replaced sutures, and most laboratory tests and diagnostic procedures will be done at home so viral diseases can be diagnosed swiftly(4). Healing and the recovery process will take place in the home or another healthful environment, since the patient will be able to be monitored by videophone and interactive television.

People will assume the major responsibility for the maintenance of their own health. Daily physical checkups will be possible, since telemedicine services will be widely available in homes or at convenient locations. There will be a wide use of computers to prescribe medications. Computers will also be used for individual psychotherapy, and group psychotherapy will be possible via videophone conference.

Emphasis in the future health care system will be placed on effective healing techniques rather than on the intrusive procedures and treatments common today. There will be a virtual cessation of medical doctors providing clinical services except for surgery. Most of medicine as we know it today will be computerized. Nursing, which has maintained caring as its very essence and central focus, cannot and will not be computerized. The nursing system will devote itself to providing guidance in self-care and to promoting self-healing by sustaining a genuine caring relationship with clients. Caring is a universal and ancient phenomenon that transcends specific cultures, time, and technologies(5).

Professional nurses will provide the primary care by serving families in their own settings. The nurse will not work in isolation, since direct communication with health information members through telecommunication technology will be widely available. Written reports and paperwork will have been replaced by dictaphone technology.

Health histories stored in data banks will be readily retrievable for analytic, diagnostic, and prognostic purposes. This information will be directly available to the client as well as to the health care professional who assists the client in sorting the data, synthesizing the available information about the current state of health, and determining a care regime based on the client's own priorities and values.

The nurse will be active in preventing emotional and psychosocial problems, since tests will be available to reliably predict the probability of an individual developing some major emotional or psychosocial problem in later years(4). Preventive medicine will also be a reality because of the advances in predictive medical techniques and the synthesis of specific antibodies.

The future will see nurses using technology to its fullest advantage both for themselves and their clients, instead of technology abusing and controlling the functions of nurses.

KOAN

In light of the above projection of the future consider the following:

If this vision of nursing and the health care system were to become a reality in your lifetime, what direct effects would it have upon you?

Would your current skills and educational experience prepare you to function independently in the system described? Or does the security of the medieval system still have its hold on you?

Has your education prepared you to focus on the process, the interrelationships, the significance, or the meaning of events rather than on the memorization of facts and isolated bits of information?

Are you prepared to assist clients to develop their own goals rather than to impose the goals established and promoted by the health professional?

Do you know as much about health and how to maintain it as about disease and its treatment?

Have your rewards come primarily from the satisfaction and approval of the client or from the approval and rewards of the system?

What nursing skills and expertise do you currently possess and/or use to enhance and promote health and healing?

Healing and health promotion in their fullest sense consist of both curing and caring. The lay healers and midwives of earlier times combined both functions successfully.

But with the development of scientific medicine, and the modern medical profession, the two functions were split irrevocably. Curing became the exclusive province of the doctor; caring was relegated to the nurse. All credit for the patient's recovery went to the doctor and his "quick fix," for only the doctor participated in the mystique of Science. The nurse's activities, on the other hand, were barely distinguishable from those of a servant. She had no power, no magic and no claim to the credit(2, p. 40).

As society becomes even more aware of the limits of medicine and the benefits of health maintenance and self-care, the balance of power could shift. Will the nursing system be ready when it does?

CATALYSTS AND BLOCKS

To 70% of all working nurses employed by hospitals today, this vision of nursing could be most unsettling. Working within the complex organizational structure of the hospital, the nurse, like Sisyphus, has many "gods" to whom she must answer—the nursing hierarchy, the administration, and the medical staff. Attempts to identify and plan for the needs of clients and patients often conflict with the demands of the system for efficiency, control, and cost-effectiveness. Realistically, the sanctions and approval of patients and clients may mean little in a system where the patient is often powerless and too weak or passive to be heard.

But what incentives exist for nurses to change the system? Nurses have always been seduced by the promise that they could humanize and individualize the care given in traditional settings. Yet, innovation in nursing care can be a double-edged sword to the innovators. The bureaucratic structure of traditional institutions and the tyranny of the medical model (see p. 205) have often thwarted the humanizing efforts of nurses. In fact, as some nurses have attempted to change and improve the quality of care in institutions, their efforts have often been labeled self-aggrandizing "power grabs."

KOAN

You have recently been involved in a public protest against a local health care institution for what you consider the institution's blatant interference

---

in the nurse's right to practice. You became very visible during the protest. You were interviewed by the media and quoted in local newspapers. You published your views in a nursing magazine. Because of your definite position on the issues, you decided to resign your position in the institution against which you were protesting.

Two months later, while attending a nursing conference, you are seated at a banquet table with some colleagues. One of your colleagues introduces you to someone at the table you had not previously met. She introduces you as "one of the nurses active in the recent protest." You smile and acknowledge the introduction. The woman looks at you and quietly exlaims, "Oh, you're one of those nurses who want all the power?"

What would be your reply?

Power and innovation are often inescapably intertwined. Nursing's power base in traditional settings, including hospitals, and in society, in general has been diluted and diffuse. Attempts by nurses to strengthen their power base in order to improve the system are often severely restricted by administrators, physicians, nurses themselves, and society. Margaret Sanger's persistent efforts, for example, to bring information about childbirth and birth control to working-class women led to her imprisonment, humiliation, and silence from her own profession. It might be well to remember that second order change agents often receive their greatest accolades posthumously. It might also be well to recognize that the greatest source of power for change exists in the public's approval of their efforts.

CURRENT HEALTH CARE DILEMMAS

The greatest innovators in nursing were sensitive to the pulse of public opinion. They were also acutely aware of the incongruities in the systems in which they worked. For example, despite the prestige of the British army and the good breeding of its gentlemen officers, the common soldier was treated like fodder in the Crimean War. Nightingale was appalled at the unsavory conditions to which the sick and wounded soldiers were subjected. With the assistance of the *London Times,* Ms. Nightingale enlightened the public, garnered public and political support, and initiated reforms that ultimately carried over into all health care. Likewise, Margaret Sanger was impressed by and sensitized to the dilemmas created by childbirth and birth control that were faced by immigrant women and their husbands who had come to America to seek opportunities to fulfill their dreams of a happy life. She worked to close the gap between the dream and the reality by bringing her case to the public. An appraisal of the dilemmas of the current health care system might further sensitize nurses to those aspects of the system that need revision and reform.

Over the last two centuries improvements in health have resulted more from improved nutrition, birth control, and sanitation than from advances in medical technology(6). In fact, West ern culture's romance with the scientific method, techniques, and hardware has overridden the fundamental objective of caring for the patient. Many people are deprived of treatment or preventive care as resources are lavished on costly, exotic equipment that, comparatively, saves few lives(7). Dimond believes that an emphasis on humanism in the current system would complement the scientific approach(8).

Only 10% of major health problems are directly affected by medical treatment today. Ninety percent of a person's health status is determined by factors related to personal health practices that are beyond the physician's control, such as eating habits, smoking, exercise habits, and the quality of air, water, food, and work environments(9). For example, for the first time in modern history more people die prematurely because they eat too much rather than too little(7, p. 44). And yet, there are sections of this country, particularly in some areas of the South, where a diversified, enriched diet would probably contribute more to the health of the population than increasing the number of hospital beds or physicians(9).

Ninety percent of the nation's medical expenditures go to cover the costs of attempts to cure or control specific illness, while less than 3% is earmarked for prevention and less than 1% for health education(9). Moreover, the effectiveness of medical care seems to decline at the same rate as costs rise. Illich asserts that while the cost of living has risen about 74% in the past 20 years, the cost of medical care has risen by 330%(9).

The public's concern over the current state of the health care system was revealed in the Harris poll of June 1978, reported at a special White House briefing(11). The results of the Harris report revealed the following dilemmas:

1. Americans want better health care for less money but are ambivalent about how to get it.
2. Consumers want a voice in health issues such as rising hospital costs, and they want the federal government to get out of the hospital management business. Americans feel a "deep distrust of what they perceive as a mindless bureaucracy."
3. Seventy percent of the respondents believe that the entire system is uncontrolled and needs change. At the same time a majority said that they were satisfied with the quality of health care.
4. Thirty percent of respondents were unhappy with both physicians and nurses' services.
5. A majority believes that higher priority should be given to preventive medicine rather than to curative medicine.
6. Responses of over 90% of the sample reflect the belief that better nutrition, less smoking or no smoking, weight control, and exercise are the most important factors in good health.

Harris believes that the time may be at hand for a major shift in priorities in health care. The new view may result in people being charged for "medical service on the basis of how much they need to go to visit doctors and hospitals. . . . This would put a premium on patients who take care of themselves so that they would pay less of the "freight" of health insurance(11, pp. 36–37). Dr. John Thompson, who helped develop the Harris survey, believes that the general public is beginning to view prevention as cost effective and beneficial even though it is "not as sexy as open-heart surgery, nor is it as exciting as new technology like CAT scanners. . . ."(11, pp. 36–37).

Health professionals, particularly nurses, are taking a dim view of the current health system, especially hospitals. A survey of nearly 17,000 nurses revealed that nurses consider hospitalization to be dangerous primarily because of understaffing(12).

1. Sixty percent of the respondents considered the hospitals in which they worked to be understaffed.
2. Twenty-one percent claimed that these hospitals were badly understaffed.
3. Twenty-three percent cited instances of dangerous conditions for patients due to understaffing, such as:
   a. One registered nurse, one licensed practical nurse, and one aide caring for 18 spinal-cord injury patients, 15 with quadriplegia, and 3 with paraplegia.
   b. One registered nurse and one aide caring for 30 to 36 postoperative patients.
   c. One registered nurse and one aide caring for 25 newborn babies, 5 of them premature.

This analysis of how nurses rate the quality of care that patients receive from nurses and doctors further revealed that physical care was rated good or excellent by 77% of the respondents, but only 32% rated psychological support of patients as being good, with the psychological support of relatives being rated even lower. While ratings on physical care were naturally related to the nature of the service (ICU requiring more physical care than psychiatry or maternity), overall the rating for psychological support given by physicians was consistently lower than the ratings for nurses. The nurse respondents to this survey see themselves as better "carers" than do physicians. "Caring" as the essence of nursing must not be sacrificed to the demands of an impersonalized health care system. The president of the AHA responded to the survey by noting that it "reflected a national problem; the geographic maldistribution of nurses and the fact that nursing manpower sources vary widely from state to state and within states"(9). He also acknowledged that cost containment exerts a growing pressure on health care, which poses difficulties for hospital administrators trying to justify increased staffing.

OBSTACLES TO CHANGE

Attitudes

The present crisis-oriented, after-the-fact medical approach to health care is costly, ineffective, and unsatisfactory. More emphasis on prevention is recognized as a better investment to improve health, increase longevity, and lower the cost of health care. The need for change is obvious, but the resistance to change is great. This is reflected in the attitudes of many health professionals.

Many physicians do not find preventive medicine financially lucrative, intellectually challenging, or personally rewarding. Some feel that prevention counseling is neither wanted nor accepted by most of their patients. Levin points out that "physicians and other health professionals may perceive that self-care poses a threat to their unusually privileged economic status, as well as to their monopolistic possession of technical knowledge"(12). Some health care professionals, both doctors and nurses with paternalistic attitudes, believe that only they possess the scientific knowledge and wisdom for proper decision-making in the management of health. Levin calls this attitude "the arbitrary and oppressive differentiation between provider and consumer"(13, p. 38). Illich claims that this attitude in the health care system actually destroys health by diminishing people's autonomous ability to cope. "By turning patients into passive consumers, objects to be repaired, voyeurs of their own treatment, the medical enterprise saps the will of the people to suffer their own reality"(10, p. 69).

The public's attitude toward the curtailment of unhealthy practices, such as excessive smoking, drinking, overeating, and inactivity, is generally negative. At the same time, the public harbors unrealistic expectations that medicine can provide rapid cure or relief for all illness. There will always be a segment of the public who wish to maintain complete dependence on health professionals, with the blind faith and belief that they know best.

The industrial manufacturers of medical technology survive on the development of costly, complicated new equipment for diagnosis and treatment. Blackburn says that twice as much is spent each year on developing an artificial heart than on the most expensive program to prevent heart disease(9).

The powerful meat, dairy, sugar, and tobacco industries resist efforts at preventive education to curtail the unhealthy consumption of their products. The lax public and professional attitude toward health education in general is a major barrier to change. Knowles claims that the school health programs have been "abysmally ineffective" and that the physician's own professional education includes very little about nutrition, which is a critical element in most of the major health problems today(9).

KOAN

Is it reasonable to expect a health care system to be all things to all people? Can it be altruistic and capitalistic at the same time? Rank the following services in order of their priority to you and then compare your rankings with those of your fellow students or colleagues.

_____ Ready access to competent medical care whenever needed on a 24-hour basis (not physician of choice).

_____ Personalized care by your own physician.

_____ A tax-based national health insurance for medical, dental, and skilled nursing care expenses.

_____ Access to well-equipped medical centers with the most advanced technology (CAT scanners, kidney dialysis).

_____ The right to collaborate in making all health care decisions pertaining to yourself.

_____ Mass screening and early disease detection programs with computer data bank storage of all health information.

The Medical Monopoly

No one can deny that medicine has held a monopoly in the health care system. The AMA lobbied hard and long for strong medical licensing laws for over 50 years. Medicine even strengthened its position in the health care system through the early nurse registration laws that institutionalized and gave public sanction to the unequal status of nurse and physician(1, pp. 115–116). The Flexner Report, which helped standardize medical practice and eliminate alternative educational models, created a guaranteed minimum quality among members of the medical profession.

Current opposition to the medical monopoly does not imply a position against individual physicians or the practice of medicine. Rather it means opposition to a system that has blocked efforts to return decision-making control to the consumer and has minimized the importance of health promotion and prevention. White, a San Francisco cancer specialist who heads the California Medical Association committee that studies evolving systems such as the holistic health movement, says, "We (the medical profession) came up with the monopoly without coming up with much evidence that our methods worked"(14). California law grants physicians a monopoly on all healing in an attempt to protect the public from charlatans and thieves; unfortunately, this category includes any of the drugless practitioners and midwives as well. Since California is the birthplace of the many holistic group movements such as the East-West Academy of the Healing Arts and the Council of Nurse Healers, it may be the testing ground for legal suits that will challenge the existing monopoly of physicians in controlling all areas of health care practice. Rick Carlson, a nonpracticing attorney who works as a consultant for government agencies and holistic health groups, believes that practitioners of alternative approaches to health care have cause for complaint against the medical monopoly(15). In addition, with the public demanding access to new practices and practitioners, the field is loosening up and a few states have even begun to dismantle the medical monopoly. An example of this is the recent legislation that allows the licensing of nurse midwives in the state of Maryland(16). Carlson advises health care practitioners to stop looking at the injustices of the past. Now is the time to devote energies to pioneering innovations for the future.

KOAN

In view of the education and experience you have already acquired, what pioneering innovation in health care might you have to offer the system?

Barriers to change must be kept in perspective while indices of changing practices are being sought and new trends are being forecast. The shifting attitude toward responsibility for one's own health is being prompted by accumulating evidence that preventive measures and health education can reduce risk of illness and early death as well as reduce health care costs. Prevention through effective public health programs designed to better living conditions, including sanitation, nutrition, immunization against infectious diseases, and birth control, have done more to improve health and control disease than all medical advances to date. Knowles claims that the American public, inspired by an unrealistic hope and medicine's own excessive claims, has been praying and paying for miracles the doctor cannot deliver(9). Medicine's monopoly of the health care system to this point has created a backdrop for the reemergence of holistic health care.

THE REEMERGENCE OF HOLISTIC HEALTH PRACTICES

Past and Present Trends

Holistic health care practices attempt to treat the mind, body, and spirit as a unified entity. Holistic health is based on the notion that the person, not the disease, is the center of focus in healing. This approach recognizes the individual as a whole—a complete organism that has qualities transcending the parts. The holistic health philosophy is an effective force toward the promotion of self-healing. It is a system that emphasizes the individual's responsibility for his or her own well-being and embraces practices from many cultures that have not been used by traditional Western medicine. Any technique, ancient or new, such as acupressure or therapeutic touch that helps to reestablish the psycho-physiological harmony and balance in the human organism is considered for use if it is safe and effective. The holistic health movement does not entirely reject the skilled techniques of modern medicine. It does, however, question the arbitrary and mechanistic stance of the medical system, which is paradoxically called a "health" care system. Although great technological strides have been made to enhance diagnostic abilities, replace worn or diseased parts, and repair devastating injury to the human organism, the inability to manage the most common chronic health problems and promote healing has been a source of embarrassment to modern medicine.

Science seems to have had little use for the concept of self-healing since the discovery of the germ theory. Healing is restoration with or without the assistance of medicine. Traditionally, medicine has not been in the forefront of movements that emphasized people's abilities to release, enhance, or restore their own healing powers. Nursing has, from its beginnings, leaned more toward the holistic health model. Nightingale cited as the primary objective of nursing to "assist the reparative process" (17). (see Table 6-1 for a comparison of the medical model and the holistic health model.)

In the early part of the nineteenth century, alternatives to orthodox medical practice gained popular support as people tried to avoid violent forms of therapy such as bloodletting and leeching. This period of American medical history was dominated by the teachings and prolific writings of Benjamin Rush, M.D., signer of the Declaration of Independence. Rush advocated the use of bloodletting, induced vomiting with drugs, purging (use of cathartics to cleanse the bowels), sweating, salivation, and cupping the skin to the point of blistering(18). His treatment regimens were based on a theory that disease was caused by an accumulation of bodily poisons that had to be eliminated even by drastic means. Medications were given in such large dosages that the result was often worse than the disease being treated. Not all his contemporaries believed in his violent system of medicine but few opposed him, since he was such a renowned patriot and so active in public affairs.

History books now acknowledge the fact that in many cases Rush's therapeutics did more harm than good. Bordley states that Rush's "treatment for Yellow Fever consisted of daily bleedings of twelve ounces or more of blood and daily purging with a mixture

Table 6–1. Differences Between the Medical Model and the Holistic Health Model[a]

Medical Model	Holistic Health Model
A deviancy will be placed within the medical model if it is seen as:	Views issues of maintaining and regaining states of health within the framework of:
1. Nonvoluntary.	1. Self-responsibility.
2. Organic (emphasizes mind-body dualism, linear causality, reductionistic theory).	2. Organismic perspective (a person as a unified whole, holistic theories emphasizing human-environment interaction.)
3. Treatable by physicians.	3. The person as the primary decision-maker, the health professional as facilitator and provider of alternatives.
4. Having disease as the primary focus.	4. Person-family-community orientation instead of disease as the primary focus.
The medical model rests on a foundation of classical Newtonian physics.	The holistic model incorporates the new physics as its basis.

[a] This table was compiled from:
1. Veatch RM: The Medical Model: its nature and problems, in *The Hastings Center Studies.* 1973, vol 1, no 3, pp 59 – 76.
2. Siegler M, Osmond H: The 'sick role' revisited, in *The Hastings Center Studies.* 1973, vol 1, no 3, pp 41 – 58.
3. Callahan D: The WHO definition of health, in *The Hastings Center Studies.* 1973, vol 1, no 3, pp 77 – 87.

of calomel and jalop (cathartics), until the patient either recovered or died. About half of his Yellow Fever patients were in the latter category"(18, p. 35). In his obstetrical practice Rush bled his patients 30 ounces at the beginning of labor and at the same time administered purgatives. Although some modifications occurred, the Rush method of medical practice continued for several decades after his death.

Credit for eroding Rush's unpopular but well-entrenched medical practices was attributed to the public opposition of William Cobbett, an English writer and politician who came to the United States in 1792(18, p. 35). He took the case before the public through his satirical writings. He was sued for libel by Rush, but Rush's court victory failed to silence Cobbett. Rush's legal victory, in fact, attracted more followers to the campaign against bleeding and purging. The Rush-Cobbett case is yet another example of public opinion prevailing over legal ruling. Cobbett continued to speak to the issues despite the risk. One wonders how many major issues are being raised and fought away from public awareness by nurses who believe that working quietly within the system will bring the needed change?

In the final analysis, opposition to Rush's violent therapeutics came not from his dissenting colleagues but from the skeptical public searching for more palliative treatments that were gentler and safer. The public's rejection of extreme medical treatment grew into what was termed the Popular Health Movement of the 1830s and 1840s.

Ehrenreich and English also attribute the Popular Health Movement to a general social upheaval stirred up by feminist and working-class movements to reestablish the lay practitioners who were being replaced by organized medicine(2, p. 24). The formally trained doctors were male, usually middle class, and almost always more expensive than their lay competitors. Physicians' formal training was of little value because of the system of medical education in this country and the absence of a body of medical science.

Lay practitioners were undoubtedly safer and more effective than the "regular" doctors, who had some degree of formal education because they relied more on "mild herbal medication, dietary changes and hand-holding rather than on the heroic interventions popularized by Benjamin Rush"(2, p. 26).

Most medical history books dismiss this period as the high tide of quackery and medical cultism. This is understandable, since the new teachings were antithetical to everything that came to be identified with traditional medical practice. For instance, women were the backbone of the movement, teaching anatomy and personal hygiene (as does the Boston Women's Health Collective of today) with an emphasis on prevention rather than on the intrusive violent medical practices of the day. Women were advocating frequent bathing (which physicians considered a vice), loose-fitting female clothing, whole-grain cereals, temperance, and even birth control(2, p. 25).

The Popular Health Movement of the 1800s represented both a class struggle and a feminist struggle, because these two forces converged in this movement. The Popular Health Movement "was not just a movement for more and better medical care, but for a radically different kind of health care. It was a substantive challenge to the prevailing medical dogma, practice and theory" (2, p. 27).

KOAN

Can you draw any parallels between the feminist involvement in the Popular Health Movement and the modern women's liberation movement and the holistic health care movement?

Many nontraditional practices flourished within the medical cults that were part of the Popular Health Movement. Some of the practices were certainly nontoxic and promoted health and healing, while others were most likely quackery. Examples of these cults are listed in Table 6-2.

As the specific cults became more popular and posed a threat to traditional medicine, medical leaders mounted campaigns to convince the public of the dangers of these unorthodox practices. The public, however, continued to support many of the less scientific but more humanistic approaches to treatment. Oliver Wendell Holmes claimed that homeopathy was effective because 90% of those patients commonly treated by a physician "would recover, sooner or later, with more or less difficulty, provided nothing were done to interfere seriously with the efforts of nature"(17, p. 44). Even though Holmes considered homeopathic medicine to be quackery, he had to admit that in 9 out of 10 cases, the weak dosage of medication interfered less with the healing powers of the body than the excessive dosages prescribed by the orthodox medical doctors.

As the Popular Health Movement began to degenerate into a set of competing sects, regular doctors were able to pull themselves together and reorganize formally into the formidable American Medical Association. The cults and practices of the

Table 6–2. Popular Health Movement Cults

Hydropathy	Advocated the avoidance of drugs and the use of various types of water for treatments and baths. Exercise, good hygiene, and a diet of natural foods were recommended.
Thomsonians	Used herbs and established several schools known as botanico-medical colleges.
Grahamites	Taught that the maintenance of good health depended on the observance of hygienic measures and a diet of natural vegetables and whole wheat flour. Graham crackers originated with the Grahamites.
Osteopathy	Substituted spinal manipulation and body massage for drugs. Osteopathic medical schools remain today.
Christian Science	Was and is based on the belief that religious faith heals. Does not advocate or permit drugs or invasive procedures.
Homeopathy	Advocated the use of minute dosages of medications rather than the massive dosages prescribed by regular doctors in the treatment of disease. Homeopathy is still practiced today.

The contents of this table were compiled from references 2 and 18.

Popular Health Movement of the 1830s and 1840s may have served as a foundation for some of the holistic health practices of today.

As science advanced in the 1800s, so did medicine's ability to diagnose and identify disease. Thus was heralded the dawn of the truly scientific approach. Traditionally medical research has focused on the physiology of disease and treatment approaches derived from data collected from research subjects who had the disease being studied. Criticism of this model centers on its narrow perspective and its after-the-fact orientation. In the recent past, researchers have awakened to the value of studying prediction and prevention. The health hazard appraisal, for example, has evolved from this prevention model, the roots of which may date from the ancient health cults of Greece and later from the cults of the Popular Health Movement.

The health hazard appraisal is a tool of prospective medicine that is currently gaining popularity as the focus shifts toward a preventative health promotion model of care(18). This tool attempts to do a quantitative assessment of the major health risks affecting individuals before the onset of illness. Risk is interpreted as the chances of a person encountering illnesses, accidents, or death-producing incidents in a lifetime. Data based on U.S. mortality figures is used for comparative information on the leading causes of death by groupings for age, race, and sex. Abridged tables have been developed to estimate the probabilities of death from all causes within a five-year span. Information on the person's lifestyle and personal health practices is then fed into a computer for a comprehensive analysis of personal risk factors. Information gleaned from the analysis is of limited value to many people unless professional counseling and guidance is given during interpretation of the results of the appraisal. Most people need assistance in relating the information to their own values and belief systems, establishing priorities in their health care practices, and determining realistic goals for changing health-related behaviors. While such tools suggest changes that are needed to maintain or regain health, the "how" is the most crucial component and depends on the knowledge and counseling skills of an empathetic, caring person such as a professional nurse.

After the person has achieved some of the recommended behavioral changes, risk reduction can be computed and repeated periodically for feedback on performance and continued assessment. The purpose of the appraisal process is to enrich and extend the span of useful life by reducing disability and death due to preventable risks. This information can help the person to become more specifically aware of the association between personal health states and such lifestyle factors as diet, degree of obesity, smoking habits, and type and amount of physical activity or exercise practiced daily. The relationship between personal health and lifestyle is presented in terms of the statistical likelihood of death in the next ten years due to any of the leading causes of death for a person's age and sex group as well as to their combined effect. This mortality risk is converted into an equivalent appraised or "physiological body" age at which the average person of the given sex has the same risk. The computerized health hazard appraisal printout then presents the extent to which the appraised risks and age could theoretically be reduced by complying with certain recommended changes in health-related behaviors.

The health hazard appraisal is a portent of the future. This tool is already being used for client assessments by nurses. It emphasizes collaboration between health care provider and health care recipient. It also emphasizes the client's role in decision-making and self-responsibility, ushering in a new era of client accountability. The health hazard appraisal is a tool not only for use by nurses in private practice, but one that can easily be integrated into the usual hospital outpatient clinic routine for assessment of potential problems of clients and into the planning of health teaching programs that can be individualized and preventive in nature. It is a tool that can also be used by the occupational health nurse to evaluate the risk potential of workers and to plan preventative programs.

The potential use of the health hazard appraisal in traditional clinical settings is just as great as its use in outpatient, HMO, and private clinic settings. The question is whether the acute care facility is willing to budget time and money to invest in preventive health programs.

THE MODERN SELF-CARE MOVEMENT

A statement in a recent medical journal described the self-care movement as "medicine's fastest rolling new bandwagon"(14, p. 30). The self-care movement is growing in popularity for many reasons. An international conference in Copenhagen in 1975 explored this social medical phenomenon and identified some of the reasons for the modern self-care movement(13, p. 20). They are listed as:

1. The "demystification" of primary medical care
2. "Consumerism" and popular demands for increased self-control related to antitechnological and antiauthority sentiments
3. Changes in lifestyle and rising educational levels
4. Lay concern with regard to perceived abuse in medical care
5. The lack of availability of professional services(13, p. 20).

In Williamsburg, Virginia, in 1734, John Tennent published his work, *Every Man His Own Doctor or The Poor Planter's Physician.*

It continued through five editions. Self-care has been an attribute of most societies and cultures through time, but its prevalence and popularity depend upon a number of social and political factors, including:

1. Public dissatisfaction with the existing system but particularly with the monopolization of the health care system by one profession powerful enough to ignore public demands or consumer wishes.
2. Scarcity of medical services in particular areas, which, ironically, fosters more independence and confidence in one's own ability to cope.
3. A shift from acute infectious diseases in the population to chronic disease and a concomitant increased cost factor(13, pp. 19–29).

The self-care movement can be either an imminent threat to health care professionals or an asset, depending upon the viewpoint of the observer. The president of the American Academy of Family Physicians said, "One of the most exciting things that's going to happen in the next 10 years will be the increasing involvement of patients in their own health care"(19). Others, more comfortable with the traditional ways of the health care system may not share the enthusiasm of this physician. In fact, some health care professionals may yearn for the patient to play his rightful role, "the sick role."

Talcott Parsons' sick role theory, published in 1951, views physicians as authority figures and patients as dependent. "Conflict or even legitimate difference of opinion is not part of this conceptualization, although a failure to comply is possible and there is a growing body of sociologic literature that addresses the phenomenon of noncompliance with the medical regime"(20). Eliot Freidson proposed another model of the patient role in light of the current state of affairs in the health system. "He sees patients and providers as occupying different positions in the social system, and indicates a clash in perspectives is not unexpected"(2).

Factors contributing to the change in the physician-patient relationship include increased consumer knowledge, increased volume of services provided, greater awareness of health needs and practices, medical specialization's replacement of the family doctor and his trust relationship with patients, and growing dissatisfaction with health care as evidenced by increasing malpractice suits.

KOAN

Have any of the above factors changed your relationships with clients/patients? How have your relationships with clients/patients been affected?

Defining Self-Care

Some of the controversy surrounding the concept of self-care centers on disagreement over definition and functions. Differences will continue to exist, since the terms *self-help, self-care, medical care,* and *health care* are used interchangeably by various groups. Two definitions presented at the Copenhagen Conference offer a foundation for viewing the self-care model. Self-care is:

1. "An action taken by the consumer or patient, to reduce, to the degree possible, incremental debilitation resulting from chronic disease"(12, p. 11).
2. "A process whereby a layperson functions on his/her own behalf in health promotion and prevention and in disease detection and treatment at the level of the primary resource in the health care system"(21).

Further clarification is provided by Fry's identification of the four major roles for self-care:

1. Health maintenance and disease prevention
2. Self-diagnosis
3. Self-medication
4. Patient participation in professional care (use of services)(12, p. 11).

These functions or roles are based on the premise that the self-care phenomenon lies outside the structure and framework of the professional health system. Self-care is voluntary, self-limited, and nonorganized. It is reflected in behaviors involving lifestyles and decision-making processes. Many studies indicate that anywhere from 75 to 90% of health care in this country is actually self-care or care undertaken by the family(9). Many traditional practices or home remedies have proven to be 90% appropriate and relevant according to studies done both in Britain and in Denmark(9). In America, "Most family doctors are badly overworked, yet half or more of their patients, by the doctor's own judgment have problems for which a physician's services are not indicated"(14, p. 39). The self-care movement continues to reveal interesting contrasts with practices in the more traditional health care system. One such contrast lies in the difference between education for self-care and patient education in the more traditional sense of the word. Since patient education, patient teaching, and health teaching (whichever terms are most familiar) are such a growing part of nursing practice, it is important to analyze the differences, proposed by Levin, between the self-care and the patient education model. Levin says "The biggest difference, perhaps, is that patient education focuses on what the professional thinks is good for the patient, whereas self-care education is determined by what the learner perceives as his needs and goals"(22, p. 170). For purposes of contrast, Levin's analysis of the differences between the two models is presented in Table 6-3.

Boundaries between the opposite positions presented in Table 6-3 may be eroding as the self-care movement evolves in conjunction with other social changes. The self-care and patient education approaches need not be in opposition. To survive they need to be mutually complimentary, as they can be if health professionals change some of their basic assumptions about the danger of self-diagnosis and self-treatment. Health professionals need to accept a new set of assumptions that acknowledge that "people's integrity in making health decisions and their ability to perform successfully on their own behalf take precedence over any and all existing professional values of risk reduction and disease cure" (22). Wider use of lay people and organized self-help groups has been hampered by the professional's reluctance to acknowledge their valuable role and the necessity for their services in the health care system. Attempts to professionalize this lay movement with standards, guidelines, techniques, or content sugges-

Table 6–3. Contrasts Between Education for Self-Care and Patient Education [a]

Self-Care	Patient Education
Motivation	
Health promotion or disease prevention (may be counterproductive to hospitals that derive major economic resources from inpatient income.	Could be income-producing or efficiency enhancing to health service. May also be motivated to prevent recurrence of specific disease.
Roles	
Well-person role (does not assume sickness.) Care means to look after.	Sick person under the "care" of another.
Educational Goals	
Goals derived from learner's perceived needs and preferences. Both content and method controlled by the lay person. Learning outcomes may not always agree with professional's health values.	Uses medical-approach focus on content not directed at reducing dependency. Major goal of teaching is optimal compliance with professionally preferred health behaviors. Control remains in hands of professional.
Content and Substance	
Prevention and protection from the assaultive diseases, those iatrogenically caused (disease caused by the treatment given). Emphasis on how to manage the professional care system.	Prevention and risk reduction from the insultive diseases and disabilities caused by biological, psychological, and environmental factors.
Knowledge Base	
Relies heavily on knowledge and skills of the consumer. Emphasizes individual as decision-maker in the goals of promotion, prevention, detection, and treatment of disease.	Assumes that learner has little or no previous knowledge of subject. Teaching designed to impart new knowledge and skills for specific conditions.
Teaching Strategies	
Educational strategies providing actual experience in gaining fundamental control over one's health destiny as well as needed skills.	Uses methods appropriate to teaching specific skills (active learner trials under supervision).

214

Table 6-3. *(Continued)*

Self-Care	Patient Education
Population	
Any self-motivated lay persons in any state of health.	Patients of traditional care-givers.
Environmental Role	
Personal health status is strongly related to environmental forces. Concern is with social change as well as reduction in personal risk factors.	Focus is on the individual's health behavior (lifestyle, diet, etc.) over which he has personal control. Very little consideration is given to socio-environmental factors.

a The major information in Table 6−3 is taken from reference 22.

tions might lead to professional dominance and a stifling of creativity. Support and resources can be offered without attempts to gain control. If professionals in the health care system resist the movement for individual determinism—for more control over one's health and choice of treatment—the self-care movement may become a powerful force against the traditional organized health care system rather than complementary to it. The fate of the modern self-care movement may then parallel the fate of the Popular Health Movement.

Nursing and the Self-Care Movement: A Possible Future

Much of nursing's efforts in patient teaching have been based on the medical model with its disease orientation, although some efforts have been truly health oriented. Lucille Kinlein, a pioneer in independent nursing practice, defines nursing as assisting in the patient's self-care practices in regard to his or her state of health(22). Kinlein struggled during her first few years of practice to delineate the differences between nursing practice and medical practice clearly, based on their divergent concepts of health. Medicine begins with the concept of disease and views health in terms of the absence or presence of disease. Nursing, Kinlein believes, must focus on the health state of the person. This health state is a continuous concern and not just a consideration during times of illness or disease. In the self-care approach "health is viewed as a natural resource, a condition to meet life goals and not a goal in itself" (Nowakowski and Valiga, unpublished article, 1978). Health in this new perspective is viewed as energy or a reservoir of strength and skills that people use to manage their lives. The emphasis is placed on self-responsibility and client control. The professional serves as a resource to assist people in formulating and meeting their own goals. Clients are supported in making health-related decisions and in developing self-care practices that promote health and maintain or regain the level of health and energy necessary to meet their life goals.

One example of the self-care movement's influence on traditional practice is the Center for Continuing Health Education at Georgetown University, founded by Dr. Sehnert. This center was an outgrowth of the standard health education classes provided for clinic patients. Sehnert recognized the need to clearly communicate to clients the nature of their health conditions. He began responding to clients' requests to be taught how to do specific procedures for themselves such as taking their own bloodpressure and interpreting the significance of the reading, administering their own allergy shots, and using the otoscope to look into their children's ears. Sehnert called his program "A Course for the Self-Activated Person." The content of his classes include instruction in the following areas:

1. Acquiring and using a black bag of medical tools, including stethoscope, blood pressure cuff, otoscope, tongue blades, high intensity penlight, dental mirror, oral and rectal thermometers.
2. Learning to pay more attention to the body's messages such as headache, sore throat, and fatigue as well as feeling good.
3. Gaining familiarity with drugs to develop kits of prescription drugs and other remedies appropriate to family needs.
4. Introductory yoga.
5. Obtaining, reading, and keeping a copy of one's own medical record.
6. Learning how to interview and rate prospective doctors or one's current physician.
7. Planning a visit to the doctor and learning how to get a busy doctor to answer questions.

8. Using decision-making charts called clinical algorithms to decide what to do when confronted with common illnesses, injuries, and emergencies(19, p. 38).

Most classes offered are patterned after this model, with variations to accommodate specific group interests and needs. Sehnert has started a movement for support of the self-care concept within the medical profession. The nurses in the Georgetown Health Education Center have proposed an educational program that differs in focus from Sehnert's original concept. In the nurses' model the "primary focus is to assist participants to develop the intellectual and emotional skills which will enable them to assume increased responsibility for self in health" (Nowakowski and Valiga, unpublished article, 1978). Meeting these objectives requires more than just skills training. The major change in emphasis of the nurses' educational program is a shift to different learning approaches in order for behavioral and value changes to occur developmentally in individuals over a period of time.

Nursing has taken an active but not always highly visible role in the self-care and holistic health movement. Not all of nursing's efforts have been publicized as much as Milio's storefront efforts in Chicago in the early 1970s(24), the Kentucky Frontier Nursing Service(25), Kinlein's independent health practice(26), or the American Nurses' Foundation project "Know Your Body"(27)—a program for early health screening and education of school-age children. In addition, numerous new groups of nurse-healers and their associates are organizing and providing support for those who are seeking alternatives to the current system. It seems that the health care system has come full circle to another holistic health movement. This new health movement, like the Popular Health Movement of the 1800s, was born out of the social and political upheavals and the rights movements of the 1960s. Levin calls this era an exciting one of transition in health care

> . . . from a professionally dominated world of service to one of self service. The process of demystifying medicine and demedicalizing society is just now rising in our consciousness as a profound turning point in the history of health. We must come to terms with changing patterns of morbidity, emerging pluralism in chronic disease care, less right and

moralistic perspective in avoidance of risk, recognition of iatrogenic effect and appreciation of the lay resources as the primary and least dangerous health resource(21, p. 175).

KOAN

Will nursing get increasingly active in the movement for reform of the health care system?

Will nursing abandon those traditional settings that are repressive and limit the potential for quality nursing care? Or will nursing attempt to challenge and change repressive systems?

Will nursing defend and support the current system relying on other levels of workers to provide nursing care?

Will nursing increasingly move into independent practice and into nontraditional settings to provide primary care?

Will nurse practice acts change to reinforce this movement?

Will nursing redefine its roles and functions in response to the needs of a changing society or will this be determined for nursing by others?

Will nursing finally abandon the medical-disease model and fully reembrace holistic health care?

THE AMBIGUOUS FUTURE—THE POTENTIAL OF AMBIGUITY

The oracle of Delphi was cryptic and vague to those who consulted her. This was an intentional maneuver so that the individual would essentially carve out the future of him- or herself based on hints given and the individual interpretation of those hints. In contemplating the future of nursing's part in the health care system, one might follow the cryptic counsel of Don Juan, the mythical Indian sage in Castanada's *Journey to Ixtlan.* In charting our course for the future,

... we only have two alternatives; we either take everything for sure and real, or we don't. If we follow the first, we end up bored to death with ourselves and with the world. If we follow the second and erase personal history, we create a fog around us, a very exciting and mysterious state in which nobody knows where the rabbit will pop out, not even ourselves.

When nothing is for sure we remain alert, perennially on our toes. . . . It is more exciting not to know which bush the rabbit is hiding behind than to behave as though we know everything(28).

REFERENCES

1. Ashley J: *Hospitals, Paternalism and the Role of the Nurse.* New York, Teachers College Press, 1976.

2. Ehrenreich B, English D: *Witches, Midwives, and Nurses: A History of Women Healers.* New York, The Feminist Press, 1973.

3. Churchman CW: Epilogue, the past's future in estimating trends by systems theory in Klih G (ed): *Trends in General Systems Theory.* New York, John Wiley & Sons, 1971, p 441.

4. Maxmen J: *The Post Physician Era: Medicine in the 21st Century.* New York, John Wiley & Sons, 1976.

5. Leininger M (ed): *Transcultural Nursing: Theories and Practice.* New York, John Wiley & Sons, 1977, pp 3–22.

6. McKeown T: Determinants of health. *Human Nature* 1:60–67, 1978.

7. Carlson RJ: Health in America: What are the prospects. *The Center Magazine* 5:43–47, 1972.

8. Dimond EG: Medicine—where it seems to be. *JAMA 238: 1251* •1255, 1977.

9. Brody JE: Specialists look to preventive medicine to improve nation's health. *New York Times* May 30, 1978, p 135.

10. Illich I: Medicine is a major threat to health. *Psychology Today,* 9:66–67, 1976.

11. Eastman M: What the public thinks about health care—according to Harris. *American Pharmacy* 518:36–37, August 1978.

12. Funkhouser R: Quality of care: Part I. *Nursing 76* 16:22–31, 1976.

13. Levin LS, Katz A, Holst E: *Self Care: Lay Initiatives in Health.* New York, Prodest, Neale Watson Academic Publications, Inc, 1976, p 20.

14. Butler K: The rise of the outlaw healers. *New Age* 3:30, 1978.

15. Kaslof LJ: *Wholistic Dimensions in Healing: A Resource Guide.* New York, Doubleday Co Inc, 1978.

16. CNM: Services are reimbursable in Maryland. *Am J Nurs* 78:1143, 1978.

17. Nightingale F: *Notes on Nursing.* London, Harrison, 1860, p 6.

18. Bordley J, McGehee H: *Two Centuries of American Medicine: 1776–1976.* Philadelphia, WB Saunders Company, 1976.

19. Davis HS, Milsum JH: Implementation of the health hazards appraisal and its impediments. *Can J Public Health* 69:227–232, 1978.

20. Ferguson T: Medical self-care, *New Age,* 3:38, 1978.

21. Bullough B: Stratification in Hardy M, Conway M (eds): *Role Theory: Perspectives for Health Professionals.* New York, Appleton-Century-Crofts, 1978, pp 157–176.

22. Levin LS: Patient education and self care: How do they differ? *Nurs Outlook.* 26:170–175, March 1978.

23. Levin LS: The lay person as the primary health care practitioner. *Public Health Rep* 91:209, 1976.

24. Kinlein L: The self care concept. *Am J Nurs* 77:601, 1977.

25. Milio N: Self care in urban settings. *Health Educ Monogr* 5:136–144, Summer 1977.

26. Dock L, Stewart I: *A Short History of Nursing.* New York, GP Putnam's Sons, 1938, p 335.

27. Kinlein L: *Independent Nursing Practice With Clients.* Philadelphia, JB Lippincott Company, 1977.

28. Nurses initiate and conduct health screening and health education program in Kansas City. *Nursing Research Report.* American Nurses Foundation 12:1, May 1977.

29. Castaneda C: *Journey to Ixtlan: The Lessons of Don Juan.* New York, Simon & Schuster Inc, 1972, p 35.

Index